WHAT TO DO
ABOUT
ATHLETIC INJURIES

WHAT TO DO ABOUT ATHLETIC INJURIES

•

Thomas D. Fahey, Ed.D.

Illustrations by Sylvia Todor

Butterick Publishing

To my brothers Pat and Dan

Library of Congress Cataloging in Publication Data

Fahey, Thomas D
  What to do about athletic injuries.

  Includes index.
  1. Sports medicine. 2. Sports—Accidents and injuries. 3. Sports—Safety measures. I. Title.
RC1210.F24   617'.1027   78-27181
ISBN 0-88421-086-3

Manufactured and printed in the United States of America. Published simultaneously in the USA and Canada.

First Printing, March, 1979
Second Printing, January, 1980
Book Design: Ron Shey

Although preventative and rehabilitative exercises generally have a positive effect on your health, they are not without risk and it is, therefore, suggested that you consult with your doctor prior to the commencement of any exercise program. The author and publisher of this book assume no responsibility or liability for injury resulting from your exercise program or any activity suggested in this book.

CONTENTS

FOREWORD

Any person who participates in recreational sports or a physical fitness program notices at one point or another that physical fitness gives a feeling of well-being and actually improves the quality of life. This is a growing benefit that increases as involvement and success in athletics increase. Sometimes, however, an exercise program is interrupted—by injury. In order to get back into the game as soon as possible you must know the basics of prevention and treatment of athletic injuries.

Dr. Fahey is a physiology expert who has prescribed exercise programs for thousands of athletes, both professional and casual. He has combined his own expertise with that of sports medicine physicians and injury rehabilitation trainers and therapists to produce a book that is full of sound advice and written in understandable language.

As a physician who treats a great many athletic injuries, I can assure you that if you thoroughly digest and apply the information presented in this book your exercise program will be less frequently interrupted and you will realize far more enjoyment from it. When you get an injury you will be able to deal with it quickly, effectively, and properly. You will, as an added benefit, save hundreds of dollars in unnecessary health care costs.

What To Do About Athletic Injuries above all fosters prevention; but it also offers the information necessary for proper evaluation and immediate first aid for those inevitable injuries when they do occur.

Martin Trieb, M.D.
Chairman, Sports Medicine Committee
California Medical Association

INTRODUCTION

Perhaps the biggest objections many people have to exercising are the aches and pains that often accompany it. It's a fact that the more hours you spend participating in sports and exercise, the more of a chance you have of sustaining some kind of injury. But injuries shouldn't force you to retire from sports prematurely. There are methods of rehabilitation and treatment you can learn that can get you back in action again quickly.

The modern techniques of sports medicine can be used to combat injuries. These techniques were at first used to patch up and rehabilitate professional athletes so they could squeeze in a few more years before finishing their careers; they can now be of great benefit to the casual sportsperson, too. The weekend athlete can use modern rehabilitation methods to minimize aches and pains and to prevent injuries from becoming more serious.

Sports medicine used to be practically an art form, practiced by only a handful of knowledgeable physicians. Today it is a science with a vast accumulation of literature and research behind it. I have attempted to compile the most up-to-date information and techniques available to help *you*—whatever your level of sports participation—deal effectively with injuries when they do occur. The book contains a minimum of scientific jargon. You'll be able to understand it and use it easily.

The book is structured so that you can read it through or just look up the material that pertains to your injury. The first three chapters explain the principles of injury prevention and rehabilitation; the remaining four chapters deal with the treatment of specific injuries.

This book is not a substitute for professional medical care. It will, however, tell you when you need to call the doctor. Most people won't need a doctor for the majority of injuries they'll encounter in sports. The book will help you distinguish between a serious injury and a relatively mild one that you can manage yourself.

If you follow the advice presented here you should have fewer athletic injuries and you will recover more rapidly from those you do get. So have fun with sports. Use your common sense and a few modern techniques and you can keep those aches and pains to a minimum.

1.
PRINCIPLES OF INJURY PREVENTION

A classic picture of Jim Otto, the great football player, appeared in my local newspaper recently. Otto is shown like a *Playboy* foldout with arrows pointing to his vast array of injuries. He had about five knee operations, crushed ribs, ankle sprains, broken bones, bruises, and contusions; in short, he was a walking athletic injury. The caption read, "But I've never been carried off the field."

Many of us feel much like Jim Otto. You may not play professional football, but there may be times when you feel like you do. It's amazing how a game of volleyball or a three-mile jog can sometimes make your body feel like you experienced Armageddon and lost. Yet, a friend of mine, sixty-year old Bob Titchnell, played pro football for fifteen years without ever sustaining an injury, and he played in the days when you took your helmet off and put it in your back pocket. Why is it that some people never seem to be hurt, while others seem to get injured all the time? Are there factors that increase your chances of injury? Can injuries be prevented?

Why Me?

I become very annoyed when I have some irritating little injury that I easily could have prevented. I can think of several instances when I pushed just a little too hard while I was tired or when I aggravated a small injury until it became a big one. I should know better. Training and sports injuries sometimes produce a "Catch-22" situation: prevention of injuries requires that you get yourself in good physical condition; but you are particularly susceptible to injury when you have pushed too hard. There is a fine line between physical conditioning and physical breakdown or injury. Certainly, factors such as physical condition, structural weakness, exercise practices, equipment, and so forth will affect your chances of injury. But your personality and emotional state may also contribute to your chances of becoming a fallen weekend warrior.

Psychologists have suggested a variety of explanations for the injury-prone individual. Dr. Steven Bramwell of the University of Washington has shown that people who are experiencing a lot of life changes are more likely to become injured. He used a psychological test that measures the stability of your life by assigning a scale of numbers to the changes you are experiencing. Losing your job or a death in the family are major life changes, while personal disagreements and weight gains are lesser life changes. Presumably, numerous life changes can decrease your concentration and increase tension. Tension and lack of concentration are cited time and time again by experts as prominent factors increasing the risk of injury. When you are anxious and preoccupied, you may develop poor body positions and posture that increase your chances of getting hurt in sports.

When I introduced a friend to skiing a few years ago, she sustained a rather unfortunate injury. While she was standing on the side of a novice slope, an out-of-control skier crashed into her, breaking her leg in three places. She was in a cast for over six months. Rehabilitating the injury was difficult, but she worked very hard and was ready to try it again the next winter. Although extremely well conditioned for skiing, she was nervous and tense when she went back on the slope. On her very first downhill run, she dislocated her knee cap. Her emotional state, not her level of physical conditioning, made her more susceptible to injury.

Personality researchers have tried to establish a relationship between subconscious motivation and injury proneness. Some see the injury-prone person as rebelling against authority or as committing unconsciously intended errors as an atonement of guilt. The injury-prone person has been characterized as somewhat unorganized and sometimes preoccupied and impulsive.

Injury-prone individuals are also sometimes thought to be seeking sympathy or looking for excuses to avoid competition. Athletic coaches almost universally recognize this phenomenon. Sometimes they go overboard and shun injured players even to the point of institutionalizing the practice. I know of one coach who established a "Hall of Shame," a list of players who were injured and unable to participate.

No doubt there are malingerers among athletes, but I think that most injuries are genuine. Examine your own motives: be honest with yourself. Are you carrying the injury bit a little too far? Are you looking for sympathy or trying to avoid having to live up to the expectations of others? If after all that soul searching you decide you have a legitimate injury, then be realistic. Work for the fastest possible rehabilitation. If, on the other hand, you decide you are really faking, then slump back in your chair and enjoy the rest.

Proneness to injury may be related to individual psychological makeup. It is certainly related to tension and anxiety. The best thing to do is take into consideration the studies, possibilities, and solid information about injury proneness. Learn about yourself and try to deal realistically with your own tendencies and psychology. Try to relax both on and off the playing field. You'll do better at your sport if you're relaxed. You'll be less likely to be injured and you'll have more fun.

Reducing the Risk of Injury

You can reduce your chances of injury if you are aware of the various situations and circumstances that increase your chances of getting hurt. Taking foolish chances and being unprepared for the inevitable are sure ways to develop problems. Learn to weigh the available options and reduce your exposure to situations where there is an increased risk of injury. Sports scientists have identified key factors involved in athletic injuries:

•*Environment.* You must first consider the playing surface. For example, if you are going to play tennis and there's water or ice on the court, try to dry the surface before playing. Running on a grass field infested with gopher holes may be asking for an ankle sprain. A ski run that you skied when the snow was packed powder may be many times more difficult when it's solid ice.

The weather conditions are important. Playing golf during a thunderstorm may turn you into a neon sign. Swimming in the ocean during heavy surf may be extremely dangerous. When you run in the rain, you must take extra precautions so that you don't fall and for getting dry when you stop.

Time of day may be important. Running on the roads during commuter hours will make you more susceptible to the effects of air pollution. Riding your bike during periods of heavy traffic may increase your chances of being hit by a car. Training at odd hours may decrease your visibility, which may in turn, increase your risk of injury. In addition, running late at night may increase your chance of being assaulted or mugged.

•*Exposure.* This refers to the role or position you are playing in a particular sport. If you are playing touch football, you are more likely to become injured if you play at an active position. A pitcher in softball is more likely to develop elbow problems than a person playing first base.

Your accumulated playing time may increase your chances of an injury. For example, if you're a golfer, it may be just a matter of time before you get hit by a stray golf ball. The more you are exposed to the situation, the more chance you have of getting hit.

 • *Physical condition.* This factor is perhaps the most important in the prevention of injuries. Your physical fitness is extremely important. Strong, flexible muscles are less likely to be injured. Try to develop a well-rounded physical fitness that prepares you for a variety of situations. If you are going to play a sport that requires rapid changes in direction, such as tennis, racquetball, or basketball, then it's not enough to prepare your body through jogging alone. Your body reacts to the stresses placed upon it. If your sport requires agility, then train for agility.

Muscle strength is perhaps the most important fitness factor protecting you against injury. However, strength is specific to particular muscles and movements. If you want to strengthen your knee joint, for example, because your sport demands great knee stability, knee extensions would be better than knee bends. Both movements exercise the leg muscles, but knee extensions develop the muscles on the inside of the thigh (vastus medialis) that are extremely important to knee stability. The best strength program, then, is one that develops your muscles in a variety of ways, and one that is aimed at preventing specific injuries.

When you're aiming for well-rounded fitness, don't overtrain. Overtraining can predispose you to serious injury. Too many people try to push themselves a little too hard when they are at the limits of their capacity. Overtraining will produce several warning signs:

1. A feeling of sluggishness
2. Poor exercise performances
3. Muscle soreness, particularly in the legs
4. Evidence of lower resistance to such problems as colds, headaches, cold sores, or general malaise

If you are suffering from overtraining, then the worst thing you can do is to train harder. This sounds obvious, but you would be surprised how many experienced and accomplished athletes ignore this principle.

Overtraining causes a depletion of the carbohydrate or sugar stores (glycogen) in your muscles and liver. Carbohydrates are the most important fuel for muscular exercise. The best way to rebuild your body's carbohydrate stores is by resting and making sure you take in enough carbohydrates in your diet. Breads, grains, fruits, and seeds are valuable sources of carbohydrates.

A present or previous injury may predispose you to worsening your disability or creating entirely new problems. Take precautions against making an existing injury worse. Don't return to your sport too early. If you do play with an injury, try to protect your body by taping the area or perhaps by using protective padding. Keep working on rehabilitating your injury even after it feels like it's better. Try to strengthen an injured area as much as you can. The stronger it is, the less chance you'll have of reinjuring it.

Fatigue may also contribute to injury. The best way to avoid fatigue is to get into good shape. However, even the best athletes in the world get tired. When you feel yourself getting too tired, stop playing. You are leaving yourself open for an injury if you go on. You have little to gain by practicing when you are fatigued. In fact, you may be hurting your game. Practicing skills when you're tired can lead to bad habits that will ultimately lead to poor performances. In addition, tired muscles may have difficulty holding your body in strong positions while you're playing. When you develop poor body mechanics, you are asking for trouble.

Drugs, including alcohol, can be a menace as far as injuries are concerned. Drugs and alcohol may impair judgment and coordination and increase your risk of injury. Drugs such as amphetamines, that are believed by some to improve performance, can disturb the body's metabolism and have led to death in several instances.

• *Equipment.* Good quality equipment is essential for preventing injuries and for enabling you to play up to your potential. You must have equipment you can count on. Basically, you get what you pay for. Those five dollar track shoes with the stripes you bought at the local bargain mart may look like the real thing, but they are probably poorly constructed and made of inferior material.

If a sport calls for protective clothing, wear it. My laboratory assistant has a bicycling helmet that makes him look like the village idiot, and I used to razz him about it every time he wore it. One day, he was in a serious accident. The only thing that prevented him from having a severe head injury was his helmet.

Even experienced sportspersons should wear protective equipment. Wear a life jacket for water sports such as water skiing, white water rafting, and boating. Wear a helmet for hard-surface sports such as skateboarding, bicycling and motorcycling, and hang-gliding. Don't be a "No-net Nanette"; wear protective clothing.

• *Rules.* Sports rules have been established, in part, to minimize the risk of injury. Some of the most serious injuries I have seen have occurred in sandlot basketball and football games where participants didn't strictly abide by the rules. There used to be a television beer commercial a few years ago that featured a mythical touch football team called the Stinson Beach Chargers. The scene was typical of any beach or park anywhere—a bunch of people getting together for an impromptu athletic contest, often blasted from numerous cans of beer. These athletic party situations carry with them a high risk of injury. Often brute force is substituted for finesse. Such games sometimes result in mayhem—and broken bones, joint dislocations, and other serious injuries. I'm not saying to avoid sandlot games—they can be a lot of fun. But do beware of injuries.

• *Body mechanics and sports techniques.* Good fundamentals and body mechanics can prevent many of the injuries you experience. In most sports it's a good idea to get some coaching, particularly when you're first learning. If you start off on the right foot, you will be less likely to develop habits that may lead to injury and poor play.

Good body mechanics means that your body is held in strong positions. Many injuries occur when you're off balance, when your body may be in an awkward position. When you have good body mechanics, you are better balanced and you can maintain a lower center of gravity. A lower center of gravity gives you more stability and makes you more prepared for the unexpected. It's the unexpected that sometimes results in injury.

Good sports techniques imply that your movements are efficient. There is little wasted effort. The end result is that you're less tired as the game progresses. You are more likely to become injured when you are tired. When fatigue sets in you lose your balance and concentration. You're susceptible to injury.

• *Experience.* The number of years of participation in a sport often has a correlation with your chances of getting hurt. When you are a beginner your movements are inefficient, you fatigue easily, and you may use poor equipment. When you become more experienced, you avoid situations that lead to injury. I'm not saying you play less aggressively, it's just that your approach becomes more effective.

In certain sports such as scuba diving and skiing there is definitely a higher injury rate among beginners, particularly among those who never had any instruction. In sports like running, you've got to learn to read your body. You learn that if you have pushed too hard one day, then you had better lay back the next day or you'll be subject to injury. You learn to wear the shoes that work best for you.

Sports savvy takes time to acquire, but you can avoid getting all of your education the hard knocks way. Read everything you can get your hands on about your sport. Talk to other people who share your sporting interests; they may have had experiences you could benefit from. Consult your local newspapers for notices of exercise clinics and sports workshops. You'll learn a lot and you'll gain a lot of experience.

• *Your age.* Injuries occur most often to young children and the older participant. Younger sportspersons generally have poorly developed muscular coordination which makes them susceptible to injury. Lack of judgment also tends to increase the occurrence of sports disabilities among younger people.

Older people tend to lose muscle flexibility. It is extremely important for an older person to regularly practice joint mobility exercises that will help prevent aches and pains and help maintain normal movement capacity.

As you get older, you have an increased risk of heart disease. You should take every precaution to assure that exercise is going to be a healthy, positive experience. Every person over thirty-five years of age should have an exercise electrocardiogram determined on a treadmill at least every two years. The treadmill test (sometimes called a stress test) is generally administered in a hospital by a cardiologist. However, special sports medicine facilities have been established throughout the country that specialize in helping you with your exercise program. These centers not only conduct treadmill stress tests, but perform detailed studies of your body fat and muscle strength and flexibility.

The treadmill test is an important prerequisite to beginning an exercise program. This stress test will tell you whether your heart is operating effectively and can give you information about optimal training levels for an exercise program. The test can help you get the most from your exercise program and will help insure that your activity program is safe. After all, exercise should be increasing your health and happiness, not turning you into an invalid.

It is particularly important that older people observe the rules of injury prevention. Warm up before exercise. Warming up should include a full battery of flexibility exercises and some easy movements similar to the movements in the sport you're going to participate in. So, if you are going to run, your warm up should include flexibility exercises and at least several minutes of fast walking and jogging. Cool down after exercise. Put your warm-up suit on and walk slowly until your body temperature has returned close to normal. One of the worst things you can do is to finish a brisk run and jump immediately into a hot shower. The hot water may send much of your blood to your skin and you may faint. Although this can happen at any age, it is particularly dangerous in older people whose circulatory systems don't react as quickly to change.

As you get older you must be particularly careful to rehabilitate injuries fully before resuming vigorous levels of activity. Your program should be progressive, that is, increase the severity gradually and in small steps. A key phrase is: "Train, don't strain." You can reach high levels of training at any age. However, when you are older, it's much easier to do too much too soon.

• *Peer-group pressure.* People will do things in a group they would never attempt by themselves. In some ways this is good. Only by pushing yourself can you ever expect to improve. However, this situation sets the stage for overdoing it. You may be goaded into doing something you're not physically capable of. You may extend yourself beyond the limits of your endurance. The result may be a serious injury.

It's a good idea to challenge yourself, but don't get carried away. Don't attempt something if it's way beyond your capacity. We are all enamored of the idea of David and Goliath. But David was lucky he didn't develop tennis elbow. Challenge yourself a little at a time. That way you will be assured of continued success with a minimum chance of injury.

• *Your own psychology.* I have already discussed the injury-prone individual. There are other phenomena that can increase the risk of injury. One of them is the "old-pro syndrome." This condition exists when physical abilities, lost for many years, still exist in the mind. I'm all for positive thinking, but there is a difference between positive attitudes and fantasy. Learn about your own capacity. Get a feel for what you are really capable of doing. That five-minute mile you ran in college may not be possible now. Redevelop your fitness gradually. You will once again be capable of high levels of performance if you consistently, but slowly, increase your fitness.

Developing Your Physical Fitness

The best thing you can do to prevent injury is get yourself in the best possible physical condition. This involves developing the specific physi-

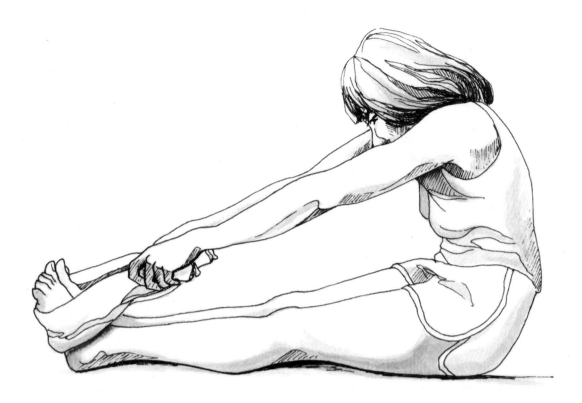

Good flexibility is important for preventing injury.

cal attributes required for the sports in which you hope to participate, as well as the basic endurance, strength, flexibility, speed, and skill required for any sport. Analyze the requirements of your sports and prepare yourself accordingly. For example, if you want to play sports that require rapid changes in direction, such as tennis or basketball, then you have to develop your speed and agility.

Overall fitness development is the subject of my book, *The Good-Time Fitness Book* (Butterick Publishing, 1978), and if you want a detailed discussion of this subject, I suggest you read it. There is a simple method, however, of determining your fitness and readiness for sports—the mets method. The mets method has been developed by numerous sports scientists over the past thirty years. What are mets? A met is the amount of energy required by your body at rest. The intensity of an exercise can be expressed in terms of the increased energy required above rest. Mets tell you how much energy is required to perform a particular exercise. At rest your energy requirement is 1 met. During exercise you need more energy than at rest so your met level is higher. The harder the exercise, the higher the met level. For example, running a six-minute mile requires 16 mets, while an eight-minute mile only requires 13 mets.

The energy cost of most sports has been determined and appears on the chart entitled Approximate Met Cost and Fitness Requirements, page 22. The mets column tells you the energy requirements of a sport or exercise. For example, the energy cost of skiing is between 5 and 8 mets. This means you must increase your metabolism 5–8 times above resting to ski. Mets tell you how hard you have to work to play a sport.

You can also use the mets chart to determine if you are in good enough physical condition to play a particular sport. The second column, "minimum max mets," refers to your maximum capacity or your physical fitness. Your max mets is the number of times you are capable of increasing your energy level above rest. It is a measure of your maximum capacity and physical fitness. The higher your max mets, the more exercise you can do. I measure max mets in my laboratory with expensive computerized equipment, but you can get a pretty good estimate of your max mets by taking the 1½-mile run test. The faster you can cover the distance, the higher your max mets. By comparing your max mets with the minimum max mets requirement of a sport, you can determine if you are in shape for the activity. For example, racquetball has an energy requirement of between 8–12 mets. If your max mets (maximum capacity) was only 10 mets, you would be exhausted within minutes. You need a higher energy capacity (max mets) than the sport requires. For racquetball you need a max mets of at least 13–14 to play comfortably. If you are in shape, you greatly reduce the chance of an injury.

Determining Your Max Mets

The 1½-mile run is used to determine your max mets. Do not take this test unless you have been running regularly for a minimum of six weeks. If you haven't been running, you must gradually prepare yourself for the test. The preparation will take between five and ten weeks. The following chart will bring you through the preparation period. Do not move from one week's level to the next until you can comfortably complete the present week's workout.

Week	Workout	Days Per Week
1	1½-miles: alternate jogging 50 yards and walking 50 yards	4
2	2 miles: alternate jogging 100 yards and walking 100 yards	5
3	2 miles: alternate jogging 300 yards and walking 100 yards	5
4	2 miles: alternate jogging 400–600 yards and walking 100 yards	4–5
5	2 miles: jog as far as you can, walk 100 yards, jog-walk the remainder of 2 miles	4–5

When you are ready for the 1½-mile run test, find a running track or a running course that you know the exact length of. Warm up first by jogging at a slow pace for several minutes. When you are ready, try to run the 1½ miles as fast as you can. You can determine your max mets from the 1½-Mile Run Test chart.

1½-MILE RUN TEST

Time Min:Sec	Your Max Mets
8:05	18.0
8:20	17.5
8:35	17.0
8:55	16.5
9:10	16.0
9:31	15.5
9:50	15.0
10:16	14.5
10:35	14.0
11:01	13.5
11:31	13.0
12:01	12.5
12:35	12.0
13:10	11.5
13:50	11.0
14:31	10.5

Time Min:Sec	Your Max Mets
15:20	10.0
16:10	9.5
17:16	9.0
18:25	8.5
19:40	8.0
21:16	7.5

Determining Your Fitness for Sports

Compare your max mets with the minimum max mets required for the sport that you're interested in. Remember, the values listed are minimum. The better condition you are in, the easier the sport will be. The met cost of each sport is an estimate, but it will give you an idea of where you stand. Prepare yourself for a sport, and you will be less likely to become injured.

APPROXIMATE MET COSTS AND FITNESS REQUIREMENTS

Sport	Mets	Minimum Max Mets
Running (6 minutes per mile)	16	17.5
Running (8 minutes per mile)	13	14.5
Swimming (2 minutes per 100 yards) (noncompetitive swimmers)	12	13.5
Swimming (3 minutes per 100 yards) (noncompetitive swimmers)	5	7.5
Bicycling (20 miles per hour)	12	13.5
Bicycling (9 miles per hour)	3.5	6
Calisthenics (conditioning exercises)	3–8	5–11
Stair climbing	4–8	6.5–11
*Mountain Sports** Downhill skiing Cruising	5–8	9–12

*Altitude must be taken into consideration. Although met cost of an activity will be the same at all elevations, the higher the altitude, the more your maximum capacity decreases. Your max mets will decrease 3% every 1,000 feet above 6,000 feet.

Sport	Mets	Minimum Max Mets
Bumps and powder	7–14	12–17
Competitive	12–16	14–18
Cross country skiing		
Recreational	6–12	11–14.5
Competitive	10–21	17–24
Mountain climbing	5–10	12.5–15
Back packing	5–11	10–14
Snow shoeing	7–14	13–16.5
Sledding	4–8	7–10
Hunting		
Small game	3–7	7–10
Big game	3–14	7–16
White water kayaking	3–8	6.5–11.5
Fly fishing	5–6	6–8.5
Ice skating	5–8	8–11.5
Snowmobiling	2–4	5–6
Motorcross	6–10	10–14
Orienteering	10–20	16–22
Horseback riding	3–8	5–11.4
Water Sports		
Scuba and skin diving	5–12	8–14
Water volleyball	3–8	5–11
Fishing		
From boat or bank	2–4	4–5.5
Big game	2–7	4–10
Water skiing	5–7	8–10
Body surfing	4–7	6.5–10
Board surfing	4–7	6.5–10
Sailing	2–5	3.5–7.5
Canoeing and rowing	3–8	5–12
Competitive Sports		
Badminton	4–9	6.5–13
Basketball		
Half court	3–9	5–13
Full court	7–12	12–14
Handball	8–12	13–14
Racquetball	8–12	13–14
Squash	8–12	13–14
Softball	3–6	5–8.5
Table Tennis	3–5	5–7

Sport	Mets	Minimum Max Mets
Tennis	4–9	7–13
Volleyball	3–6	5–8.5
Gymnastics	3–5	5–7
Social Sports		
Boogie dancing	3–8	5–11.5
Square dancing	3–7	5–10
Golf		
Power cart	2–3	4–5
Walking	4–7	7–10
Roller skating	5–8	8–11.5
Horseshoes	2–3	4–5
Shuffleboard	2–3	4–5
Archery	3–4	5–6
Bowling	2–4	4–6

Developing All-Round Fitness

Endurance is important in most sports. However, other types of fitness such as strength, speed, agility, flexibility, and skill may be equally important. Work on the components of fitness necessary for your sport. Work on your weaknesses as well as your strengths. Work out a well-rounded training program and stick to it. To gain high levels of fitness you have to progress slowly but steadily. Few people are born with super abilities. You can become physically fit by diligently adhering to your program. Make sure your program is systematic—continuous work will help you develop a body capable of better performance and one that's resistant to injury. You have to educate yourself about exercise—read everything you can get your hands on. The process of developing a fit, healthy body is easy—if, you know what you're doing.

Instant Replay

    ●Certain personality factors may make you more susceptible to injury.

    ●Factors to be considered in the prevention of injury include: environment, exposure, physical condition, equipment, rules, coaching, experience, age, peer-group pressure, and psychology.

●You can prevent athletic injuries by getting in the best possible physical condition. Make sure you are prepared for the particular demands of the sport.

●Mets tell you the energy cost of a sport. Mets are a measure of exercise intensity—they tell you the amount of energy above rest required to perform a physical task. If a sport has a mets requirement of 5, that means that you must increase your energy level 5 times above rest to participate safely and successfully in it. This chapter includes a mets chart (page 22) that will tell you the energy cost of a sport.

●Your max mets are the maximum number of times you can increase your energy level above rest. Max mets tell you your highest energy level. You can determine your max mets by taking the 1½-mile run test or by taking a treadmill test in a sports medicine laboratory or hospital.

●By comparing your max mets to the mets cost of a sport, you can determine if you are physically prepared for that sport.

2.

PLAYING WITH SMALL HURTS

"**D**octor, my elbow is killing me," said Mary, with a pained expression on her face. "It hurts whenever I try to do anything with it. You've got to help me."

"Have you been doing something that might have caused the problem?" asked the doctor.

"Well, I play a lot of tennis."

"Then the answer is simple—stop playing tennis."

The doctor took a very common-sense approach to Mary's tennis elbow. By eliminating the source of the irritation, the problem would disappear. Although this is a possible alternative, Mary would have to give up playing tennis. There is a compromise solution to a situation like this. If Mary could rehabilitate her elbow using modern scientific techniques of sports medicine, she could continue to play tennis and at the same time minimize the pain in her elbow.

Most physicians are relatively unfamiliar with athletic injuries. They are usually used to dealing with disease in people who possess a minimal health status rather than people seeking high levels of performance. In the past five years, we have literally gone from a nation of spectators to a nation of participants. *Newsweek* magazine has estimated that over 50 million people are engaged in a regular exercise program. People who a few years before would only see their physician for colds or serious traumatic injuries such as broken bones, are now seeking help for an array of sometimes exotic athletic injuries. Patients now seek high levels of health and physical performance. Freedom from disease is not enough. Maximal performance with a minimum of aches and pains is now the order of the day.

These new demands put physicians in a difficult position. Many doctors are not familiar with all of the injuries that occur with sports participation. Little is even known about some sports-related difficulties. Often the injuries are not problems at all, but simply transient aches and pains that develop during physical conditioning. Minor problems can be a drag on a doctor's time, preventing attention to more important cases. People involved in sports need to take some responsibility for their own health care, and to be able to recognize the difference between a serious problem requiring professional help and a problem they can successfully deal with themselves.

Doctors can treat the symptoms of your sports-related pain. They may be able to give you a pill to relax a muscle in spasm or a brace to help protect an injured joint. However, only you can manage the long-term treatment and rehabilitation of your injury. Only you can strengthen and increase the flexibility of a body part that's been injured. What you need is the knowledge of when to rest and when to work a little harder. You need to be able to distinguish between a pain that's relatively normal and part of the training process and a pain that's serious and requires medical attention.

Taking Responsibility for Yourself

Pain is a very personal thing. It's almost impossible to measure. Individual differences in pain tolerance make the guidelines for professional consultation difficult to establish. For example, an orthopedic surgeon I know compared two of his recent patients—one a weekend runner and the other a professional soccer player. He performed knee surgery on both. He could find nothing wrong with the runner's knee. It looked completely functional and could have caused only relatively minor discomfort. The soccer player's knee was a mess. The surgeon was amazed at his ability to walk let alone play soccer, but who is to say that the runner was not in great pain?

You must learn to assess the status of your body accurately. There are differences between naturally occurring short-lived aches and pains of sport and more serious long term injuries. This knowledge comes with experience and a systematic development of knowledge of the principles of injury prevention.

In order to take some responsibility for your own health care, you must take every precaution against becoming injured, and when you are injured, take steps to insure that the problem doesn't get worse. There are some specific steps you can take to prevent injuries and minimize their effects when they do occur.

• *Stay in shape.* You can prevent injuries from occurring if you are in the best possible physical condition. Weak and inflexible muscles are easily injured. Many joints in your body are supported and protected by muscle. To fortify your joints, these muscles should be as strong and dynamically functional as possible. People who are out of shape become injured much more easily than the physically fit. The unconditioned people easily exceed their capacity—and fatigue is the mother of injury. The physically fit person fatigues less easily. Physical fitness means not only general conditioning, but being prepared for the specific demands of the sport. If a sport calls for upper body strength, it's not enough to be able to run an eight-minute mile. Fitness requires the development of endurance, strength, flexibility, speed, and skill. The more fit you become, the less chance you have of becoming injured.

• *Warm up before you exercise.* Your joints and muscles are less susceptible to injury when they are warmed up. Your warm up should include stretching and slow movements similar to those you're going to do in your sport. Your heart needs to be warmed up too. Avoid high speed movements until you are warmed up. Start off slow, gradually increasing the speed. Warming up becomes particularly important as you get older. There is a tendency for the body to become less flexible with age. Be sure to warm up as part of any sports activity.

• *Don't let your muscles get cold.* Warm muscles are less prone to injury. Chilled muscles are more susceptible to spasm and injury. When you are finished exercising, put on something dry and stay out of drafts. Wear a sweat suit when you are standing around. If you have been in the cold after exercising and plan to exercise again shortly, be sure to repeat your warm-up procedure. It's easy to tighten up after physical activity. During periods of rest after exercise, try to keep moving—even if it is just a slow walk. Avoid exercising when you're cold.

• *Get good equipment that's suited to you.* Sports are challenging enough without your being handicapped by poor equipment that makes you more prone to injury. For example, using cheap running shoes may cause foot problems that will plague you for many months. Inexpensive ski bindings may cause you to break your leg. On the other hand, don't use equipment designed for a professional athlete—a tennis racquet strung too tight for your ability and strength may cause you to develop tennis elbow. Buy shoes that are made for the sport. Jogging shoes are inappropriate for tennis and racquetball and vice versa.

If a sport calls for protective equipment, wear it. I went white water river rafting a few years ago and decided I didn't need a life jacket. I felt it was too bulky. The raft flipped and I was lucky I didn't drown. If people would only wear protective gear, the number of injuries could be cut down dramatically.

• *When you get soft tissue injury, use ice, compression, and elevation if possible.* Soft tissue injuries, injuries to muscles and joints, are often accompanied by swelling. Rapid recovery requires keeping the swelling to a minimum. The old standby, the hot bath, may be the worst thing because it promotes swelling. Ice therapy has been shown to retard swelling and to deaden the pain that accompanies injury. Elevation and

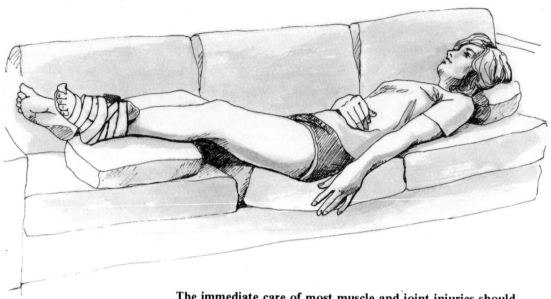

The immediate care of most muscle and joint injuries should include ice, compression, elevation, and rest.

compression of injuries with an elastic bandage will also help minimize swelling.

•*Rest and immobilization is often necessary when you become injured.* The classic remedy of the traditional coach was "run it off." This doesn't always work. Don't underestimate an injury. A minor complaint can become a major problem if you keep aggravating the situation. Sometimes rest is the best solution, but in many cases you don't have to become bedridden or even sedentary. A running injury may not be aggravated in a swimming pool or on a bicycle. Using alternative training methods, you can maintain your physical fitness level without making your injury worse.

Sometimes you just have to let nature take its course. Overmotivated "weekend warriors" can sometimes make a situation worse by pushing too hard. Sometimes rest is the best remedy.

•*Rehabilitate that injury slowly but steadily.* This is where you are really in the driver's seat. You can have the best sports medicine physician available helping you and still never recover from an injury if you don't follow this principle. Remember, Marcus Welby is a myth—your doctor doesn't have time to see if you are faithfully doing your strength and flexibility exercises. It's up to you. You may have injured a part of your body that wasn't in such good shape in the first place. The secret of rehabilitation is to slowly and gradually increase the strength and flexibility of the injured part.

One common mistake even top athletes make is to end the rehabilative process prematurely. They stop corrective exercise before the injury is healed. The result is a weak link that is easily reinjured. In my laboratory, I have sophisticated muscle testing devices to measure muscle weaknesses. I have found that people with muscle groups not fully rehabilitated after an injury almost invariably become reinjured.

The older you are the more important complete rehabilitation becomes. Older people tend to lose their flexibility and are more susceptible to injury. Injury often causes the formation of adhesions in your joints which tend to make you less flexible and make you even more apt to get injured. Adhesions occur when joint connective tissue sticks together. Work on your flexibility every day after an injury and you will be less prone to reinjury.

Athletic Injuries and Your Doctor

Jim moved in for a shot under the basket, exploding through two defenders. He went up, pushed the ball toward the hoop then started down, his body off balance. He landed on the side of his foot with his ankle crumpling underneath him. He collapsed to the ground in pain and was helped off the court. Then he limped home and slumped into a nice hot bath. By this time, his ankle had swelled to the size of a small watermelon. He stayed in bed for several days thinking the ankle would get better. "After all, it was only a sprain. It'll get better in a few days." The ankle didn't get better, and Jim was forced to see his doctor. It turned out that he had broken his ankle and the delay in treatment was going to make the recovery take that much longer.

Don't underestimate an injury. Whenever you sustain an injury that might be serious, you should see your doctor. If a minor injury doesn't get better, you should also seek professional help. The injury may have subtle causes that only an expert can determine.

Individual interpretation of an injury is often difficult. As a nonprofessional athlete, you can usually take a conservative approach to treating your disability. It would be pretty ridiculous for you to have a pain killer injected into your injured knee so you can finish your tennis match or your weekend touch football game. Your best bet with an apparently nonserious injury is to take it easy for a few days and see if it gets any better. If it doesn't, see your doctor to make sure that nothing is seriously wrong.

Educating yourself about injuries commonly encountered in your sport will help you assess the status of your aches and pains. With experience you will learn to differentiate between common and uncommon symptoms associated with the sport. Ask other people in the sport about their experiences with injuries. Ask a professional such as a coach or physical education teacher to share their knowledge of the problem. Attend exercise clinics. These sessions are useful for obtaining information and for meeting other people involved in the sport.

Ultimately, you are the judge of when you need to see a doctor. Be realistic. You don't need professional help if you are suffering transient aches and pains that normally accompany exercise training. On the other hand, the macho, bite-the-bullet philosophy can be overdone. Learn about sports injuries. With some problems, your doctor will be able to give you little help other than sympathy. However, the management of other problems can only be handled by a professional.

How do I Choose a Physician?

If you are looking for a physician to help you with sports-related problems, it's best to get a doctor who understands exercise. Medical schools spend little time dealing with exercise physiology or athletic injuries. I have found that the most knowledgeable sports medicine physicians are involved in sports themselves. They jog or play tennis and are generally sports oriented. They can relate their medical experience to the unique problems encountered in sports and physical exercise.

Sports injuries are often different than those typically encountered by the average physician. Most medical problems involve disease or sudden injuries. Athletes and sportspeople have presented the physician with a new category of problems: the overuse syndrome. Injuries are often caused by overusing a body part. The sportsperson is concerned about maximum health and performance. Freedom from pain is not enough. A pulled hamstring doesn't hurt when you're sitting in a chair, but it does hurt when you're sprinting across a tennis court. As an active person you need a physician who understands this distinction.

Ask active people for a physician they recommend. Word gets around. There are physicians who know a lot about sports and athletic injuries. They can help you play with small hurts. Often the team physician of a local college or high school is a good bet. Your local medical society may be able to steer you to a doctor interested in sports.

The Four Categories of Athletic Injuries

There are four basic types of athletic injuries:

- *Sudden traumatic injuries.* Examples of this are a lump caused by a blow to the head by a baseball, or a skiing accident that results in a broken bone. These injuries are sudden, and the problem is usually obvious.

- *Repeated traumatic injuries.* An example of this type of injury is a boxer being hit in the head many times.

  Bunions, which are bumps on the side of the foot, are sometimes caused by repeated trauma. If you wear shoes that don't fit, you may develop bunions because of the repeated irritation. The bunion develops out of the body's desire to protect itself.

- *Overuse injuries.* These injuries result from overworking a relatively weak area and improper sports techniques. Tennis elbow is an example of an overuse injury. Modern training methods have resulted in a rash of this type of injury. Today, even "fun runners" are putting in more than 70 miles a week. Often there is inadequate preparation or buildup for these difficult exercise programs. Overuse injuries can be tricky to deal with, particularly because the ultimate responsibility for rehabilitation lies with the individual. Your doctor can put a cast on a broken leg, but it's up to you to rest a sore Achilles tendon and take the steps to relieve the pain.

- *Imbalance injuries.* Injuries of this type are caused by such factors as poor posture, training that overdevelops some muscle groups at the expense of others, and anatomical weaknesses.

  When you use your body normally with normal movements, you don't expose yourself to injury. However, sports by their very nature involve stretching a little further or trying a little harder. By seeking excellence, you run the risk of pushing yourself too hard and exceeding your body's capacity. When you add such factors as fatigue, anxiety, anger, poor body mechanics, and bad luck, injuries may be inevitable. The trick is to prepare yourself as much as possible and not to let those aches and pains defeat you.

Posture is something many of us pay little attention to. The human body is an engineering marvel. The spine, for example, has characteristic curves that enable you to maintain an erect posture and have a lot of mobility. At the same time these curves act to absorb shock and also serve as a balance mechanism so you don't have to use much muscle power to support your body structure. When you have bad posture, you are upsetting the balance of this structure. For example, if you constantly droop your head forward, your neck muscles are called upon for support. This may lead to fatigue, tightness, and injury. Slouching in your chair may cause your back to hurt.

Muscle imbalances often cause injuries. Some people, for example, often develop the muscles on the front of the legs (quadriceps) and not the muscles on the back of the legs (hamstrings). This causes an imbalance that may result in hamstring pulls. In fact, in leg muscle testing I've done in my laboratory, I rarely see a person with injured hamstring muscles who doesn't show this type of muscle-group imbalance. Back pains are also sometimes caused by muscle weaknesses and imbalances. Back trouble is usually accompanied by weak stomach and leg muscles and inflexible hamstring and back muscles.

Man's upright posture has resulted in many aches and pains that four-legged animals don't have. Many of us have minor anatomical abnormalities that throw our bodies out of balance and increase the risk of injury. For example, if one of your legs is longer than the other, you may develop problems such as back, knee, and hip pains. Morton's toe, a pre-existing condition where one of the bones in your foot is too short, may disturb balance and result in injury.

Problems Common to Most Athletic Activities

In sports you are subject to a variety of aches and pains in your joints and muscles caused by injury, irritation, or inflammation. In this book we are more concerned about relatively minor but extremely irritating problems that may not require emergency medical attention but might still prevent you from enjoying exercise and sports at the level you would like. Specific sports seem to cause particular types of injuries, but there are problems that are common to most activities.

●*Muscle strains.* Strains are tears in the muscle–tendon complex. Tendons are tissue that hold muscle to bone. Tendons blend in with the connective tissue that holds muscles together. Strains may be relatively mild, or they can be severe, as in a completely severed Achilles tendon.

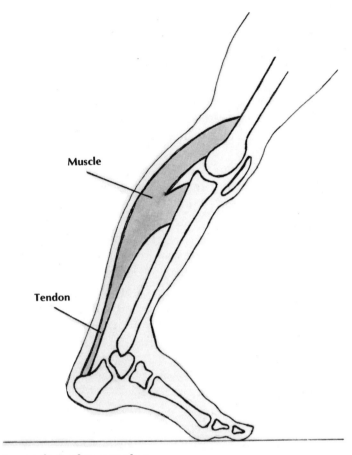

A muscle-tendon complex

Strains are very common, particularly in activities requiring rapid movements and sudden changes in direction. A pulled hamstring is an example of a strain. You have to be careful with this type of injury. Returning to activity too early can result in more serious injury.

• *Muscle spasms.* Muscle spasms are uncontrolled, painful muscle contractions that accompany many injuries. Spasms and cramps occur when your muscles' chemical system becomes upset. Although the exact causes are unknown, scientists suspect that they are related to imbalances in substances called electrolytes, such as sodium, potassium, magnesium, and calcium. Cramps may occur due to dehydration and electrolyte changes caused by exercise and/or exposure to hot environments.

• *Sprains.* Sprains result from a tear in a ligament. Ligaments are tissues that hold bones to bones. The most common sprains occur in the ankle and knee. They are potentially serious problems that often require medical attention. A serious ligament tear may require immobilization and casting, and in some cases, surgery.

• *Tendonitis.* Tendonitis is an inflammation of the tendon covering. Achilles tendonitis is an example of this type of injury. The tendon sheath becomes inflamed and causes pain. Overuse is a common cause of this kind of disability. Recovery requires rest with gentle stretching accompanied by ice therapy. Patience is absolutely necessary with tendonitis. This type of injury may take a long time to heal or become chronic if you don't deal with it effectively.

• *Contusion.* Contusions result from falls or from blows such as getting hit by a softball in the leg. There may be damage to blood vessels and muscle. These tissues may be crushed and a hematoma may form. A hematoma is clotted blood in the area of the injury. A bruise may form in the area of the injury. The contusion may also be accompanied by swelling and stiffness. Again, ice is the best treatment. A serious contusion may take a long time to heal. If the condition does not clear up within six weeks, you may have developed a calcium deposit—see your doctor.

• *Bursitis.* Bursa are closed sacs containing fluid. They are situated in areas of the body where a lot of friction or shock occurs. They are found throughout the body and are easily and often subjected to the overuse injuries common in exercise and athletics. The bursa in the heel of your foot is a common site for this type of inflammation. Treatment involves ice, rest, and protecting the area, if possible, with pads.

• *Stress fractures.* A stress fracture is a hairline break in the bone caused by overuse. These were often encountered in the feet of soldiers and were called march fractures. People involved in a lot of exercise, encounter stress fractures in the bones of the lower leg, the tibia and fibula. They can be mistaken for shin splints and are often difficult to pick up on an x-ray. Your physician may elect to put a cast on your leg as part of your treatment. In any event, you shouldn't resume training until the bone heals.

• *Skin injuries.* These include abrasions, lacerations, puncture wounds, blisters, and sunburn. These injuries can be extremely irritating and can be potentially dangerous if not treated properly.

• *Serious injuries.* Serious traumatic injuries are beyond the scope of this book. You shouldn't assume the responsibility for treating serious traumatic injury. For example a neck or head injury could result in death to the stricken person if it is handled improperly. However, I feel everyone should take the basic Red Cross courses in first aid and cardiopulmonary resuscitation.

Instant Replay

●Modern techniques of sports medicine and rehabilitation may enable you to continue playing your sport even with small hurts and at the same time get rid of those aches and pains.

●Try to choose a physician who knows something about sports and exercise. Your physician must understand that you are interested in maximal performance without injury in addition to freedom from disease.

●You must take some responsibility for your own health care. Only by keeping in good shape, getting enough rest, developing good training and technique fundamentals, and using good equipment can you expect to keep your athletic injuries to a minimum. If you develop a good knowledge of injury prevention and treatment, you can help to better manage your personal health care program.

●Follow the general principles of injury prevention and rehabilitation:

1. Stay in shape
2. Warm up before you exercise
3. Don't let your muscles get cold
4. Get good equipment that's suited to you
5. When you get a soft tissue injury, use ice, compression, and elevation if possible
6. Rest is often necessary
7. Rehabilitate that injury slowly but steadily

●The four basic categories of athletic injuries are sudden trauma, repeated trauma, overuse, and imbalance.

●Specific examples of athletic injuries include muscle strains, sprains, muscle spasms, tendonitis, contusions, bursitis, stress fractures, skin injuries, and serious injuries.

3.

REHABILITATION OF MUSCLE AND JOINT INJURIES

In the past two years, two of my friends have undergone two very similar knee operations. One, Gail, was physically active and was highly motivated to become completely rehabilitated. She was a four-times-a-week tennis player and hated the time she was laid up and unable to play. She made up her mind she was going to get back on the court as soon as possible.

After the operation, her leg was in a cast. Her doctor instructed her first to try to contract her muscles and then gradually to attempt to lift her leg off of the bed. Moving the leg was extremely difficult. Finally, after excruciating pain, she was able to pick up her leg a few inches above the mattress. She thought to herself, "I'll never get out of bed, let alone play tennis." But she kept at it. Within a few days she could lift her leg a couple of feet, and a few days later she could even walk a little with her cast on.

I introduced Gail to Frank Egenhoff, a physical therapist and a former athletic trainer with a professional football team. Frank had set up a private practice and encouraged Gail to get a prescription from her doctor for physical therapy.

When the cast finally came off, her knee looked like a mess. It was swollen and had an ugly incision that looked like a crooked railroad track. Frank started the treatment by giving her an ice massage. Gail's knee grew numb as Frank rubbed the ice directly on her oversized knee. This made the knee a little less painful. He tried to move her leg a little. After a while the knee started to warm up and began to hurt again. Frank iced the knee some more and gently tried to increase the movement in Gail's leg.

Frank began strengthening her knee. He first tested the muscle strength of the weakened limb. He used a space-age tool of sports medicine called a Cybex. The leg was only about forty percent as strong as her good leg. She had a long way to go. Frank gave her an exercise program similar to that used to rehabilitate pro-football players. The program was tough. It took almost two hours and included ice massages before and after the workout. Gail worked hard, never missing one of her three-times-a-week therapy sessions. Within a couple of months she was jogging. Six months later she had almost forgotten she had a knee operation. She was back on the tennis court, playing better and more vigorously than ever before.

Scott, my other injured friend, wasn't so lucky. Although he enjoyed sports, he was basically lazy. He was very involved in his work as a stockbroker. He found it difficult to spend much time working on his knee. After the operation he was in much pain, so he tried to follow his doctor's orders and do some leg exercises. He was progressing normally from his surgery, and after six weeks the cast was removed. He started by trying to walk on his leg. Progress was slow. He was anxious to get back to work. After a while he could get around pretty well, but his knee hurt a lot and he had a limp. With time the limp went away and he was back at work. He didn't do his knee exercises very often; after a while, he didn't do them at all.

Before his operation Scott jogged two or three times a week. It helped keep his weight down and relax him. Now he didn't jog anymore—it hurt his knee too much. The pounds started to pile on. This aggravated his sore knee a great deal, since he was requiring a weakened leg to support increased body weight. Scott no longer participated in any of the sports he liked before the surgery—he didn't want to hurt his knee. Scott had virtually become a cripple.

Two years later Gail is completely rehabilitated. She's glad she had the operation. She hasn't felt better in years. Scott, on the other hand, is bitter. He blames his orthopedic surgeon for botching the job. In a way it was his surgeon's fault. He should have encouraged Scott to rehabilitate the knee as much as possible. Too many orthopedics consider their job completed after the last stitch is sewn. The rehabilitation is just as important as the surgery, however. The injured part has got to be strengthened if it is ever to function normally again. Rehabilitation of an injury takes time, energy, and commitment.

Even minor injuries can become serious if not cared for properly. You can't take the chance that someone is going to look after you when you get hurt. Most of the responsibility for injury rehabilitation lies with you. Proper management of your injured body requires that you know such things as: when to use ice and when to use heat; how to strengthen injured muscles; how to increase a joint's range of motion, how to use tape to protect a joint, and general training procedures which facilitate the recovery from an injury.

Immediate Care of Muscle and Joint Injuries

You will very likely deal with muscle and joint injuries such as sprains, strains, and contusions yourself. Orthopedic specialists that I consulted indicated that people should "wait and see" before consulting a physician for most muscle and joint injuries. It's difficult to list hard and fast rules for separating serious from relatively benign athletic injuries, but there are some general guidelines:

- Overuse injuries such as tennis elbow, Achilles tendon pains, and sore muscles usually respond to rest and conservative rehabilitation procedures. If you get no relief from pain after several weeks, then consider seeing your physician. If these problems are relatively minor, they can be a drain on your doctor's time.
- See your doctor for head and eye injuries (except those that are obviously minor), traumatic injuries to joints that result in swelling (particularly the ankle and knee), injuries involving ligament damage (ligaments hold bones together), broken bones, and internally-related disorders such as chest pain, fainting, and intolerance to the heat.
- Listen to your body. If the pain is unbearable, then seek medical help. However, if you are experiencing muscle spasms from overexertion, there is little your doctor can really do for you. Consider the circumstances of the injury—a back injury sustained by crashing into a tree while skiing may require an x-ray while a backache caused by a vigorous golf swing may not.

You should begin rehabilitating an athletic injury as soon as you get it. First you need to immobilize the injured part. Don't try to run it off. You can easily make things worse if you run on a sprained ankle or continue lifting weights with an injured shoulder. Rest the injured part. Ice it as soon as possible. (Several techniques of icing that are most effective begin on page 48.) Elevate the injury, preferably above the heart. This will help keep the swelling down. Compress the area with an elastic bandage. Remember, elastic bandages are for compression and not for support. They provide little muscle reinforcement. Tape or braces are much more effective for support. Aspirin may be helpful for reducing inflammation and pain. In summary, the immediate care of your injury involves immobilization, ice, elevation, and compression. Rehabilitation begins with good first aid.

Recovering from an Injury

The first exercises you do following an injury should be aimed at maintaining range of motion. You will get more out of your exercises if you precede them with ice massage to the injured area. You can begin heat treatment after any swelling has disappeared. When most of the pain is gone, begin strength exercises. The stronger your muscles are, the less the risk of injury or reinjury. But work gradually, because weakened muscles are easily reinjured if pushed too far too soon.

Range of Motion

Maintaining movement capacity should be one of your first concerns. Maintenance of range of motion begins with the first aid procedures and continues throughout the reconditioning and rehabilitation period. After an injury, muscles and joints often tense up and joint adhesions form. Adhesions are fibrous tissues that make the connective tissue of your injured joint stick together. Adhesions make movement difficult and painful. Your body is attempting to keep you from making the injury worse. However, if your movements are restricted, you will lose strength and endurance that will easily subject you to further and more serious injury. To a large extent, your activities determine your flexibility. When you're injured and you have pain, your flexibility naturally tends to decrease.

The nervous system is probably the most important factor determining your flexibility. Your muscles, joints, tendons, and ligaments have a very prolific nerve supply. Special nerves called stretch receptors tell your muscles how far they're being stretched. Stretch receptors are important in protecting your muscles from being stretched too far. They are involved in the balance that must exist in body movements. They also aid in the contraction–relaxation cycle of muscles.

When stretching an injured muscle, you have to consider its biology and the way it operates.

- Ice the injured muscles before and after stretching.
- Increase the range of motion of injured muscles gradually. Overdoing this kind of exercise leads to further injury.
- Don't bounce when you stretch. Bouncing may cause small tears in your muscles or make existing tears worse. Bouncing may stimulate the stretch receptors causing your muscles to tighten up. Your stretching movements should be done gently and gradually. Flinging-type stretching exercises may also result in stretch tears that appear in or below the skin.
- Relax as much as possible during stretching exercises. There is a direct relationship between your state of mind and muscle tension.

When you have an injury, there is a natural tendency to be tense. Relax and try to forget about your hurts.

●Stretch until you feel a noticeable pulling in your muscles. Hold that position for fifteen to thirty seconds. Relax and then repeat the exercise. The ice massage will help you stretch further without as much pain.

●Don't cheat on your exercises. Do them exactly the way I describe them. Don't overstretch. As soon as you feel pain, hold it; don't try to stretch beyond that point until the pain subsides.

Strength

Strengthening injured muscles is a prerequisite to regaining speed and endurance. You should begin strength exercises as soon as most of your normal range of motion returns. Too often an injured sportsperson will try to return to tennis or jogging when an ankle hasn't recovered its strength, only to be injured again. Regaining strength requires concentrated effort. Sometimes strengthening an injured muscle group requires special equipment available only at a gymnasium. If you are serious about restoring your exercise capacity, make every effort to gain access to the correct equipment. I know of many injured sportspeople who become injured but never recover. They don't spend the twenty dollars required for a one-month membership at a gymnasium where they could use the equipment they need. These same people would think nothing of spending $200 for a pair of skis or $75 for a new tennis racquet. If you look around, you may even locate a high school, college, or recreation department whose equipment you can use free of charge.

There are many methods of strengthening an injured part of the body. These methods can be divided into four basic categories:

●Isometric
●Constant resistance
●Variable resistance
●Constant speed

Isometric exercise is muscle contraction without movement. Isometrics are the first type of strength exercise you should do following an injury. Initially, you will simply tighten the muscles of the injured area. For example, if you injure your knee, your first strengthening exercises will be composed of tightening your leg muscles. You tighten the muscles—relax—then tighten them again. Repeat this process throughout the day. You have to be careful with isometrics. It's possible to cause muscle injuries if you overdo this type of exercise.

Constant resistance exercises involve moving a weight against the forces of gravity. The resistance could be a barbell or dumbbell, or it could be your own body weight. When strengthening an injured area, the constant resistance should initially be the weight of your own body. For a knee injury, this may be simply lifting your leg from your bed. The weight of your leg serves as the resistance.

There is a vast variety of constant resistance equipment available. Included are barbells, dumbbells, knee extension and flexion machines, and weighted boots. If you sustain an ankle, knee, or hip injury, it might be a good investment to purchase weighted boots. They fasten on to your shoes and allow you to strengthen weakened leg muscles. You can order them from almost any sports store.

If you require strength equipment and you don't own any, it's probably better to join a well-equipped gymnasium. Such gyms have a large variety of equipment that the average person couldn't afford to purchase. There are now many gymnasiums that specialize in rehabilitating athletic injuries. These facilities have physical therapists on the staff who are experienced with sports-related disabilities.

Variable resistance training is relatively new and provides methods of gaining strength that were formerly unavailable. Variable resistance employs exercise machines, such as those manufactured by Nautilus and Universal Gym, to produce uniform resistance during the entire exercise. Training methods developed for these machines enable an increase in muscle endurance as well as muscle strength to occur. Many of these machines exercise very specific muscle groups, which makes them very valuable in rehabilitating a variety of muscle and joint injuries.

Constant speed exercise is also called isokinetics. Isokinetic machines are one of the most important developments in injury rehabilitation in many years. Rather than provide a constant resistance that can overwhelm an injured joint, the machine works by dictating a constant speed. The harder you push, the more resistance you feel. No matter how hard you push against the machine, the speed stays the same. The advantage of this system is that it's difficult to exceed the capacity of your injured muscles and joints. It is more difficult to worsen your disability by attempting something you're not capable of doing. Examples of isokinetic exercise machines are Cybex and Orthotron. These exercise machines have attachments that allow you to exercise many areas of the body including the ankle.

When trying to increase your strength following an injury, you should follow certain principles.

● Use ice massage before and after your exercise session. If you include flexibility exercises in a session, then you need to ice only before and after the combined training.

● Begin gradually. When injured you are particularly vulnerable to further injury.

● Warm up before you begin vigorous strength exercises. Perform the exercise with a minimal resistance before really going at it.

● Increased strength results from consistently working a little harder than before. This is the overload principle.

● Continue your strength rehabilitation exercises until you have recovered. You may experience periods when you feel pretty good and yet you may still be weak from the injury. Keep working until you are at least as good as you were before. Preferably, you should try to be stronger than you were. Your lack of strength in your legs or shoulders may be what caused you to become injured in the first place.

● Women don't develop large muscles from strength training exercises. Male hormones are required for large muscle development, so women increase their muscle size more slowly. Strength is a type of fitness that many women don't consider important. Lack of muscle strength is an important predisposing factor to athletic injuries.

Endurance

Muscle endurance is often neglected during injury rehabilitation. Dr. David Costill director of the Human Performance Laboratory at Ball State University, has found that injured muscles lose their strength and endurance rapidly after an injury. He has studied the chemical systems within muscles that are responsible for exercise performance and found that muscle enzymes react differently to strength than to endurance exercises. If you do strength exercises exclusively, the enzymes necessary for endurance will not be developed. Rehabilitating an injured area requires flexibility, strength, and endurance exercises.

If you jogged or played tennis on the moon you probably wouldn't ever develop athletic injuries. Down here on earth we have the forces of gravity to contend with. Gravity occasionally overloads our body structure beyond its capacity. The result is injury.

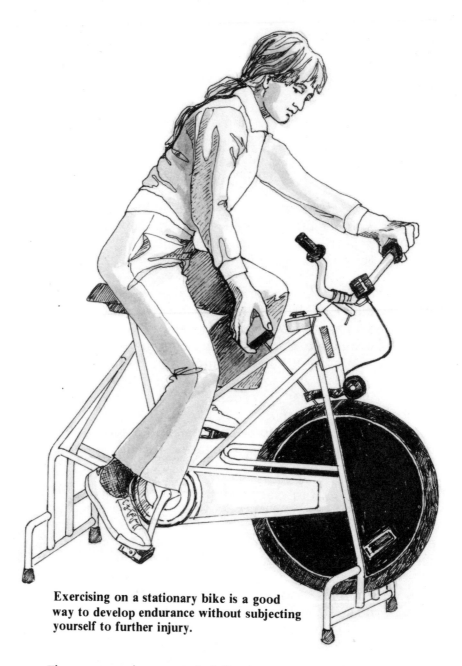

**Exercising on a stationary bike is a good
way to develop endurance without subjecting
yourself to further injury.**

There are endurance rehabilitation exercises that at least partially remove gravity from the picture. For example, you weigh no more than a few pounds in the water. In fact, space scientists conduct many of their weightlessness experiments in water. If you sustain an injury running or playing racquetball or tennis, you can maintain much of your endurance in the swimming pool. You can get a good workout without making your injury worse.

Water exercises can include much more than just swimming. You can run in the shallow end of the pool (or the deep end if you're tall) and not be subjected to the same forces of gravity present on the track. In addition, you will find stretching exercises a lot easier to do in the water. You will be amazed to see exercises that are excruciatingly painful in the gymnasium become effortless in the water. Exercising in the water will help you recover faster and give you the confidence necessary to continue your rehabilitation.

A stationary bicycle can also provide a means of getting some endurance exercise without a lot of weight bearing. This kind of exercise is boring to some people but is a means of providing conditioning without making an injury worse.

Returning to Athletic Participation

Die-hard sportspersons hate to be injured. They yearn to return to the tennis court or ski slope. You must have patience or your convalescence will be longer than you planned.

●Don't return to your sport until your injured area is restored to its full range of motion—both passively and actively. It's not just a matter of being able to move your knee, shoulder, or elbow in a nonactive situation. Your body should be able to stand the rigors of the sport in an active fashion.

●Your normal strength and power should be restored. Check the injured side of your body against the uninjured side. For example, is that injured leg the same size as the uninjured one? If not, you need more work before returning to play.

●You should have normal-coordinated patterns of movement, with all injury-compensating movement patterns, such as limping, eliminated. If you have a lower body injury, you should not only be able to run in a straight line, but also run laterally and be capable of starting and stopping rapidly.

●You should be relatively pain free. Don't expect too much. Some pain is a natural part of an active lifestyle. However, if the injured area is exceedingly painful, it hasn't healed completely.

Rehabilitation Aids

Ice Therapy

Icing an injury is one of the most important things you can do to promote a speedy recovery. Ice has the effect of reducing pain by slowing down the activity of the nerves that send pain messages. Ice relaxes the muscle and reduces spasms that usually accompany injury. Ice also helps increase the blood flow deep in the tissue without causing swelling.

One of the most important breakthroughs in the treatment of athletic injuries has been the development of cryokinetics. This involves moving an injured part after initially cooling the area with ice. In the past, the immediate treatment of an injury involved immobilization followed by heat treatment and massage. Cryokinetics still requires minimizing weight-bearing movement, but an attempt is made at maintaining the range of motion. For example, if you sprained an ankle, you would apply an ice pack, wrap it in an elastic bandage, and elevate your foot. In addition, you would attempt to move your foot up and down—first point your toes downward, then upward toward your shin. You have taken the weight off your ankle, but you are attempting to maintain the range of motion.

Ice acts as a mild anesthetic, blocking much of the pain. By using ice you can move the area. However, because all of the pain sensations are not completely eliminated, you avoid the possibility of overdoing it and making the injury worse.

The purpose of continued use of ice therapy is to regain full range of motion and normal use of your body. By reducing the pain and spasm that accompany injury, you can prevent much of the deconditioning that can occur.

The first few minutes of ice therapy will be painful; you just have to bite the bullet—this phase will pass. After several minutes, you will feel a warming sensation. Finally, the area will become numb and red. When you have reached the numb stage, you are ready to begin the rehabilitation exercises. Initially these may include easy stretching and exercises designed to restore normal range of motion. Later, they may include strength exercises and running, cycling, or swimming. Ice therapy can be used before, after, and during rehabilitation exercises. As the effects of the ice start to wear off and pain returns, the ice therapy can be repeated.

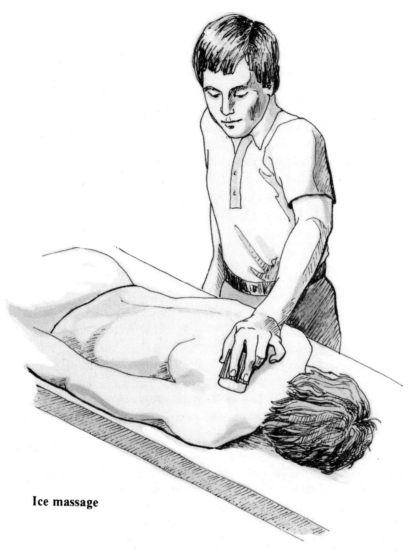

Ice massage

Ice therapy is rapidly becoming accepted by leading physicians, physical therapists, and athletic trainers. This should be one of your first lines of defense in your treatment of athletic injuries. A word of caution: never use dry ice.

Ice therapy can be used in three forms:

- Ice pack
- Ice massage
- Ice bath

An ice pack is valuable for immediate treatment. The best way to make an ice pack is to take a wet towel and put a layer of crushed ice on it. Then wrap or place the towel directly on the injury, having the ice in contact with the skin. Don't leave the pack on for too long because of the danger of frostbite. Many people put ice in a plastic bag and then place it directly on the injury. This procedure is better than nothing, but you may not be cooling the area as effectively as you could be. There are commercially available ice packs in sporting goods stores that you can put in your bag in case of emergencies. They have the benefit of being inactive until they are needed. To use them you break a chemical container that's inside the pack. This results in a chemical reaction that creates a cold pack that lasts for about twenty to thirty minutes.

The ice massage is extremely effective for focusing the cooling on a particular sport. Fill a paper cup with water and freeze it. When the ice is ready, tear away the top part of the cup and hold it by the paper on the bottom. Massage the injured part with the ice in a circular motion for about seven to ten minutes or until the part is numb. If you find that your fingers get too cold, put a tongue depressor in the cup when you make the ice. This will create a large frozen lollipop with a handle to hold on to. Peel off the whole cup.

Ice water immersion may be effective for ankles, hands, feet, elbows, and sometimes knees. This method can be used during the later stages of rehabilitation when it's no longer necessary to elevate the injured part to reduce swelling. Fill up your sink or a large basin with water, and then put in about fifteen to twenty-five ice cubes. Let the water get ice cold. Put the injured part in the water and leave it there. At first you may be able to stand only a few minutes. Take it out of the water, and then after a minute or so, put it back in. Leave it in the water for about seven or eight minutes. It probably won't do any good to keep the injured part in the water more than ten minutes. If you remain in the water too long, thirty minutes or so, you risk developing frostbite.

Heat

Heat can be used effectively after the swelling has stopped. Heat is valuable for increasing circulation and relaxing your muscles. It's probably not a good idea to use heat until about forty-eight to seventy-two hours after the injury occurred. Some authorities now recommend that you use only ice during the rehabilitation process. Remember, the rehabilitation process begins as soon as the injury occurs.

Effective healing cannot progress until there is a decrease in swelling. Heat may actually increase swelling. I know of several instances when people soaked their swollen sprained ankle in a hot tub only to make the injury much worse. Many athletic injuries involving muscle pulls, joint damage, or bruises are usually accompanied by damage to blood vessels. Heat increases swelling when this type of damage is present.

Heat can be very effective in relaxing muscles and reducing muscle spasms. After a tough game of tennis or a vigorous day of skiing, a hot tub can be very relaxing. At Mammoth Mountain ski area in southeastern California there is a natural hot spring close to the slopes. After a hard day on the slopes, it's a tradition to go down to the hot creek and settle down with a glass of your favorite wine. Very relaxing.

Wet heat seems to be the most effective. You can purchase very effective hydrocollator packs at a drug store. These are made of silicon wrapped in canvas. Heat the packs in water (do not boil—this will destroy the silicone inside), wrap them in three to seven layers of towels, then place the packs on the area that needs to be heated up. The packs are constructed to stay hot for a long time.

The authors of *How to be Your Own Doctor—Sometimes* (Grosset & Dunlap, Inc., 1976) have a good suggestion for a wet heat generator. Soak a large towel in warm water, wring it out, and then place the towel around the injured area. Cover the towel with several layers of plastic. Cover the plastic with an electric heating pad, making sure there's no contact with the wet towel. By plugging in a radio in the same socket as the heating pad, you can protect yourself from becoming French fried. The radio will crackle if the heating pad is getting wet—so, listen closely and choose a station with little static.

Other sources of relaxing heat are hot baths, whirlpools, steam rooms, saunas, and heat lamps. Be very careful. If you stand up suddenly after sitting in a hot tub, you may faint. The heat has the effect of channeling much of the blood to the skin. By standing, you suddenly make it difficult for blood to return to your heart. Blood may be momentarily cut off from your brain. There have been cases of people drowning after fainting in hot whirlpool baths.

Whirlpools should be kept at a temperature of between 90 and 112° F with 105° F being comfortable for most people. Be careful not to use a whirlpool hot bath if you've lost your tactile sense; you may be susceptible to burns. Hot whirlpools are also not a good idea if you have heart disease, fever, poor peripheral circulation, or blood clots in your legs (thrombophlebitis). Check with your doctor if you're not sure if the whirlpool is safe for you.

Contrast baths are sometimes useful in treating injuries. This treatment consists of alternating between hot and cold treatments. They are another means of stimulating circulation to injured muscles. An example would be immersion in a hot or warm bath for three to four minutes followed by a cold bath for three to four minutes. Repeat this procedure four to six times.

Heat lamps may help relax your muscles. Make sure you're using an infrared rather than an ultraviolet lamp because ultraviolet, or sunlamps, can cause severe burns in a matter of five or ten minutes. You will not be aware of the damage until several hours later. A sunlamp can even cause severe eye damage if you don't wear protective goggles. Infrared heating helps, to some extent, to increase circulation in the skin around an injured area. It may be helpful in aiding you with massage and stretching exercises. Too much of the heat lamp, however, can also cause skin irritation and burning. Don't use heat lamps over scarred, abrased, or broken skin.

The Hot Sock and Heating Lotions

You can always tell when you are around a bunch of jocks: there's always the smell of eucalyptus or wintergreen permeating the air. Injured sports people are always rubbing some sort of liniment on their aching bodies. Heating lotions are called analgesic balms and are available at any supermarket or drug store. Although it's not known exactly how these lotions work, it's believed that by mildly irritating the skin, they serve as a mild anesthetic which blocks muscles spasm and pain.

You can increase the effectiveness of the heating lotion by wrapping the area with an elastic bandage after application. An old remedy for shin splints or tennis elbow is to apply the lotion and then surround the area with a neoprene sleeve. You can purchase or construct your own sleeve with neoprene available at a scuba diving shop. The same procedure is sometimes helpful for bad backs. I should point out, however, that although neoprene "belly bands" may help your sore back, they are useless for helping you lose fat. All they do is make you sweat more.

Generally, I think heating lotions are of limited value. For some people they may cause skin irritation that may be worse than the original injury. However, they may make you feel a little better and probably won't do you any harm.

Massage

Massage is the manipulation of your muscles for the purpose of relaxation. There are few pleasures in the world more relaxing than a back rub after a hard workout. Massage can be helpful for relaxation, reduction of swelling, and increasing the range of motion. Massage may be helpful in preventing injury in a healthy person about to play a game by providing relaxation.

There are many types of massage. The hands are the most common tool and perhaps the most effective. Other tools include whirlpool air jets and vibrating machines, each of which produces its own characteristic sensation. Be aware that massage can sometimes be harmful. Massage can spread an existing infection. It can also aggravate a recent injury and actually increase swelling. It's best to wait several days after an injury before using this procedure. If the area is bruised, wait ten days before using massage.

In order to give an effective massage, you will need to use a lubricant. Something like mineral oil is probably the best. This will make your hands slide effortlessly over the skin and prevent you from irritating your subject. Make sure the person is comfortable and relaxed. Be confident; a good massage requires that you really get into the process.

There are many types of massage procedures. Briefly, they include light and deep stroking (effleurage), kneading (petrissage), friction, cupping and hacking, and vibration. Don't get overenthusiastic. If you overdo massage, you can make an injury worse. Be firm, but not harsh. I suggest you read an authoritative book on massage such as Francis Tappan's *Massage Techniques* (Macmillan Co., 1964) if you want to develop effective techniques.

Pain Blocking by Machines

An increased knowledge of our nervous system has resulted in improved methods of dealing with pain caused by athletic injuries. Pain is used to protect your body after an injury. Many times, however, you feel pain but your injury isn't severe enough to require a limitation of your activities. The pain from a mild back or ankle sprain or a sore shoulder may be irritating enough to hurt your exercise performance and interfere with the enjoyment of your sport, but if you rest the injured part too long, you will lose your physical conditioning and subject yourself to even more severe injury. Pain specialists have developed a machine that helps many people to decrease the pain they experience from many

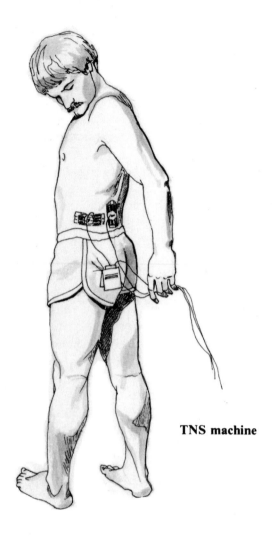

TNS machine

types of muscle and skeletal injuries. The machine is called a transcutaneous electrical nerve stimulator, or TNS.

The TNS unit is portable and can be worn comfortably during exercise. It consists of a small battery operated electrical stimulator and two electrode pads. When you turn the unit on, you electrically stimulate the part of your body that's giving you pain. This has the effect of blocking some or all of the pain sensations being sent to the brain. It's used by many professional football teams, and it could be very helpful to the more casual sportsperson as well. The TNS unit is safe, portable, and relatively inexpensive. You need a doctor's prescription to use one.

Taping

Taping techniques are the bread and butter of the athletic trainer. A kind of mystique surrounds the person who produces athletic mummies in the locker rooms of the world. Taping methods are practically passed down from one generation of trainers to the next. If you learn a few basic techniques, you can share the methods that have kept the injured immortals of sport on the playing field. Tape can be used to support injured ligaments and joints and can be used to maintain bone and joint alignment. A good tape job is almost an art form. If you are sloppy, you may leave exposed skin in an area subjected to a lot of friction. If you wrap the tape too tightly, you may decrease the circulation to your injury, thus making the pain even worse. If you wrap the injury too lightly, you provide little support. An effective tape job requires experience. However, if you start with the basics, mastering the actual taping procedures will be that much easier.

Don't buy cheap tape. Inexpensive tape provides little support and will lose its integrity when you start to exercise and perspire. I suggest you buy your supply of tape at a sports store that supplies local high schools and colleges. Grocery or drug stores often sell tape in narrow widths and the quality is open inappropriate for the heavy demands of sports.

Protect your skin before you apply tape. If applied directly, tape may irritate your skin. Shave any hairs from the area to be taped; this will save you a lot of grief when you take the tape off. You can protect your skin by applying a commercially available skin toughener before taping. In addition, various types of underwraps—thin layered polyester-urethane foam (from a sports store), panty hose, gauze, or a stocking—are available to make the taping process easier. If you use an underwrap you don't need to shave the area.

Tearing tape is an important skill to learn. Learn to tear the tape rapidly and straight: pull a length of tape from the roll; hold the roll of tape with your right hand, your right thumb anchoring the edge of the tape to the spool; using a scissors motion, tear the tape rapidly and cleanly with your left hand. If you are tearing several pieces of tape, put each piece in a place where it won't stick to the others. Be careful not to allow the tape to crimp. This happens easily, particularly when you're working with large strips.

Use the tape width appropriate to the injured part of the body. Use narrow tape for smaller, more difficult to work with areas such as the hands and feet. Areas with a large surface area such as the thighs or back need a larger width tape. It's a good idea to carry several widths of tape in your athletic bag. Athletic tape, in fact, is one of the most useful substances created by man. I have used it for everything from repairing a broken baseball bat or tennis racquet to temporarily fastening snow tire chains.

Following are the most important principles for applying tape:

•When reinforcing a joint, prevent it from going toward the direction of the injury. Taping should allow for movement but prevent reinjury. This principle is very important. Many taping procedures lose their supporting properties after about fifteen minutes of activity. Make sure your tape job is doing what it's intended to do.

•Overlap adjacent strips of tape. Don't try to save tape by sparse application. The few cents you save on an inadequate taping won't be worth it if you develop a blister from exposed skin in between tape strips.

•Avoid wrapping tape continuously. It's better to apply tape in shorter lengths. Continuous wrapping invites the risk of applying the tape too tightly, and tight taping can be very painful.

•Smooth and mold the tape as you lay it on the skin. This saves time and increases the effectiveness of your tape application. Allow the tape to follow the natural contour of the skin. If you don't, the tape will crimp and wrinkle and may pull at the skin.

Removing the tape can be unpleasant. You can use tape scissors to assist you. These have a blunt nose and can be purchased in any drug store. When removing the tape, be firm—tearing the tape in small steps only prolongs the agony.

Don't put too much reliance on taping. Sports scientists have determined that much of the benefit of tape is psychological once you have begun to exercise since movement causes your tape application to lose much of its effectiveness. When you get an injury, rehabilitate it, and it will cease to be an injury. Don't let taping become a crutch and an alternative to rehabilitation.

Braces

Various types of braces are available for injured joints. As a rule, effective braces overly restrict movement and may hamper athletic performance so, again, make every effort to rehabilitate your injury so that you won't need a brace.

Many varieties of commercially available elastic wraps are designed to reinforce your ankles, knees, elbows, and wrists. These devices, mistakenly used as braces, do little except perhaps to absorb sweat. You are much better off using adhesive tape applied directly to the skin as a brace. Elastic wraps are most effectively used to prevent swelling and should be used as part of the first aid procedures after an injury—not as a brace.

Many exotic varieties of knee braces are available. The basic types of knee braces include wraparound, hinged, ribbed, and derotation. You should use one of these braces only on the advice of an orthopedic specialist. Using an inappropriate or inadequate knee brace may give you a false sense of security. There is no substitute for strong leg muscles. At the laboratory we have found that most people are extremely weak in their lower body. This is a leading factor that accounts for the disproportionate number of knee and ankle injuries in sports. With strong leg muscles, you won't need a knee brace.

Back pain is common, particularly among more casual exercisers. Weak stomach and back muscles certainly contribute to the problem. There are many commercially available back braces. The more support they provide the more movement they restrict. Neoprene belly bands, made from material you can purchase at a scuba diving store, have been found effective for back support. They provide support and warmth and yet allow a considerable amount of movement. The major disadvantage is they cause a lot of sweating which may be a little uncomfortable.

Padding

You should use padding to protect areas that have been injured and are subjected to repeated abuse. For example, if you get a bad scrape and play a sport that subjects you to more scrapes, pad and protect the injured area. You can purchase commercially available pads for many parts of your body. If you use a little imagination, you can think of novel uses of pads designed for other sports. For example, a shin pad designed for soccer may help you protect your shins when using weight lifting knee extension machines in the local gymnasium.

Orthotics

The use of orthotics, or foot supports that place the foot in a more functional position, is receiving an increasing number of advocates among experts in sports medicine. Some injuries are caused by inherent weaknesses and structural abnormalities. In some instances, the use of orthotic devices has been shown to improve injuries such as shin splints, and to decrease knee, hip, and back pain. Sports sometimes accentuate the effects of minor structural abnormalities. Minor deviations in body structure that wouldn't effect a sedentary person at all can result in chronic pain in the jogger or tennis player.

Orthotics attempt to increase the balance and movement efficiency of the lower body. They are built from plaster casts taken of your feet. They vary in type from the soft and flexible—appropriate for sports requiring rapid changes of direction, such as tennis—to the very rigid, appropriate for forward movement sports, such as jogging or skiing.

Many runners have found that inner soles for jogging shoes increase comfort. Buy inner soles at a sports store that carries accessories appropriate for sports. Inner soles designed for walking may not hold up very well under the rigors of vigorous training.

Instant Replay

• Rehabilitation from athletic injuries requires personal commitment and hard work.

• The first line of defense against muscle and joint injuries is ice, compression, elevation, and rest from the sport.

• Rehabilitation exercises should improve strength, flexibility, and endurance.

• Criteria for return to full athletic participation are:

1. Full range of motion in the joint—both actively and passively
2. Normal strength and balance between muscles
3. Normal coordinated patterns of movement, with all injury compensation movement patterns, such as limping, eliminated
4. Relative freedom from pain

• Ice acts as a mild anesthetic and allows you to begin rehabilitation exercises earlier. It also reduces swelling and muscle spasm.

• Taping is an important procedure for reinforcing injured ligaments.

• Heat should not be used until the swelling has subsided.

• Analgesic balms are minimally effective in dealing with injuries.

●Massage is a good technique for promoting relaxation but should be used sparingly when swelling or infection is present.

●Transcutaneous electrical nerve simulators (TNS machines) have been used effectively for blocking pain sensations to the brain.

●Orthotics are used to correct anatomic abnormalities in the foot.

4.

LOWER BODY INJURIES

Lower body injuries are the most common disabilities encountered by the recreational athlete. They range in severity from sore muscles to dislocated joints and broken bones. If you maintain your interest in sports long enough, you will probably sustain some kind of leg injury eventually. The trick is to keep injuries minor and return to sports quickly.

Your legs are vulnerable to injury. They are designed to provide you with mobility while keeping you in an upright posture. Legs can generate tremendous forces that sometimes even their own structure is unable to tolerate. For example, if you kick too hard playing touch football or pivot too vigorously during a game of racquetball, you can easily sustain a knee injury. Running with unconditioned legs on pavement will usually result in shin splints. You can prevent leg injuries if you maintain a high level of physical fitness and avoid taking unnecessary chances; and, when you do become injured, keep the disability from becoming serious by following the principles of injury rehabilitation.

Lower body injuries are sometimes difficult to deal with because we are so dependent upon our legs for movement. Recovering from leg injuries requires patience and a knowledge of proper treatment. In this chapter I'll cover specific lower body injuries and how to deal with them effectively.

Leg Pains from Overuse

Overuse injuries are on the rise recently because many people have increased the severity of their training programs. A few years ago a two-mile jog was considered a long distance training program. Now that distance is a mere warm up to the thousands who have taken up road racing and marathon running.

Recently a man and woman came to me for advice on running their first marathon which was scheduled for four weeks after our meeting. They were very excited about the prospects of their new distance-run lifestyle. I tested them on a treadmill and found them to be tremendously out of shape. "What kind of running program have you been on?" I asked.

"We've been running a mile a day for the past two weeks." they said. "How do you think we'll do in the big race?"

"You people must be crazy. You'll be lucky if you can crawl home from that marathon. A race like that takes many months of preparation.

Without proper preparation, you'll both get injured. You are not ready for a marathon!"

They were disappointed. I gave them a detailed training program designed to prepare them for a 26-mile run in about eight months to a year.

Too many people get overenthusiastic and want too much too soon, or get caught up in the macho of Herculean fitness. Train in a jogging program that suits your level of fitness. From a health standpoint, there is no evidence that a marathon runner has more protection against heart disease than a person who runs two to three miles a day. In fact, marathoners are more susceptible to injury than the more casual jogger since they subject their body to so much more overuse. From an enjoyment standpoint, you're much better off playing a variety of sports rather than killing yourself a couple of hours every day on the roads. If you enjoy marathon running, then by all means continue. But prevent serious injuries by being physically prepared for the rigors of distance running. Injuries aren't fun. If you don't really see yourself as a distance runner, play some sports you enjoy.

A variety of leg pains can result from doing a little too much exercise. Overuse-related leg problems fall into these general categories:

- Overtraining
- Shin splints
- Stress fractures
- Achilles tendonitis
- Osgood–Schlatter disease

Overtraining

Overtraining is a general term for a condition resulting mainly from a depletion of carbohydrate fuel stores, or glycogen, in your muscles and liver. Glycogen is the most important fuel for high intensity exercise. Regular, heavy workouts tend to drain your muscles of this important energy source. Without enough muscle glycogen, your legs may ache and feel like lead when you try to run. Many people try to train even harder when they get in this situation. The result, even more glycogen depletion.

The best prevention and treatment for overtraining is rest and an adequate carbohydrate content in the diet. Take a few days off—when you come back, you'll feel like King Kong. You should make sure your diet contains about 70 percent carbohydrates when you're involved in heavy training such as running more than thirty or forty miles a week.

Overtraining can lead to more specific overuse injuries such as shin splints and Achilles tendonitis. There are a few general procedures to follow when you deal with this type of disability. You should rest from the activity that's causing the problem. If you have been getting shin splints from running, ride a bicycle or swim instead for a week or so. This way you will give your injury a chance to heal while you lose little of your physical conditioning. When you resume the activity, begin gradually. Gear the intensity of your training to the way you feel. Individuals heal at different rates. Don't try to work too hard too soon, or you'll only reinjure yourself. Be sure to make an effort to rehabilitate the injury before you resume training (see Chapter 3). Leg injuries sometimes take a long time to disappear. If you don't treat them patiently and consistently, you will develop a chronic injury that may take many months to heal. Obviously, something caused you to be injured in the first place. You may have been running or playing tennis in the wrong shoes; had weak, inflexible, or out of balance muscles; or you may have been running on a hard surface. Try to correct what's wrong. Finally, watch carefully for a recurrence of the injury. Often a problem will disappear only to return in a few weeks. If it does recur, consider your options—either take a more conservative approach or seek medical advice.

Shin Splints and Stress Fractures

Because of their similar symptoms and causes, I will discuss shin splints and stress fractures together. Shin splints refer to pains in the front of the lower leg. In this injury the muscles are pulled away from the bone. Stress fractures are actual damage to bone tissue. They are caused by the bone's inability to cope with the load placed upon it. Stress fractures are difficult to detect on an x-ray, sometimes not appearing until three or four weeks after the injury. Stress fractures usually project a pain that feels deep in the shin with a specific location that hurts when you touch it. Stress fractures take longer to heal than shin splints, but their treatment is similar. If shin pains do not clear up in three to four weeks, see an orthopedic specialist.

Shin splints have several probable causes:

- Overtraining when you are poorly conditioned or suddenly increasing the distance you run in a training program
  - Running or playing on a hard surface
  - Anatomical abnormalities of the foot
  - Strength and flexibility imbalances in lower leg muscles

Shin splints are common in people beginning a training program. It's important to condition yourself gradually. People who haven't exercised for years should usually start out by walking before beginning a running program. As a rule of thumb, you shouldn't start a jogging program until you can walk three miles in forty-five minutes or less. Be careful about sudden increases in training intensity even if you're in good condition. Going from a two-mile a day to a ten-mile a day running program may be devastating to your body. Increase the intensity of your workout gradually.

Hard running surfaces often cause shin splints. When you are beginning a running program especially, try to train as much as possible on grass. Playing basketball on cement at a playground may also produce leg pains when you're not in good condition. One thing you can do to combat hard surfaces is to buy good shoes. Shoe companies manufacture shoes especially designed for running on cement. They provide more padding and have soles designed to absorb shock. Insoles, that you can purchase at a sporting goods store, may also prevent shock from hard surfaces.

Anatomic abnormalities of the foot may be the subtle cause of shin splints and a variety of other foot and leg problems. A podiatrist may be able to design orthotics, special foot supports, to help clear up the problem. You might try some commercially available arch supports first. They are a lot cheaper than orthotics and for some people seem to work just fine.

Shin splints have also been associated with strength and/or flexibility imbalances in the muscles of the lower leg. You should develop the muscles in the back as well as the front of the leg. There are several exercises that may end your shin splint problems on page 65.

Treatment for shin splints includes the following:

- Ice massage the painful area (see page 48). It is particularly important to use ice after doing rehabilitation exercises.
- Rest the injured leg. Try doing some alternative nonweight-bearing exercises such as swimming or bike riding.

•Do shin and Achilles tendon stretching exercises. Do these exercises statically, that is, hold the stretch for ten seconds or so. Repeat several times.

Achilles tendon stretch

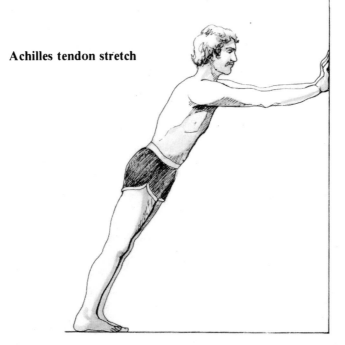

ACHILLES TENDON STRETCH Stand about three to four feet from a wall or post. Lean forward so that you're at an angle and your heels are raised. Gently push your heels toward the ground.

SHIN STRETCH In a kneeling position, toes straight back, gently sit back on your heels, pressing the tops of your feet to the ground.

•Do shin and calf muscle strengthening exercises.

SHIN EXERCISE Have someone hold your toes down. Try to pull your toes toward your shins.

CALF EXERCISES Raise up on your toes, hold that position, then relax. This exercise is even more effective if you do it with weights on your shoulders, or with calf strengthening machines available at a gymnasium.

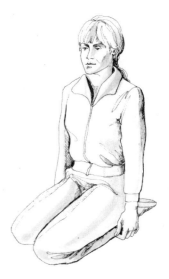

Shin stretch

●If you are overweight, lose a few pounds. This will place less of a load on your sore leg muscles.

●Return to activity gradually, making sure to train on soft surfaces.

●Aspirin may help relieve the pain.

●If the condition persists for more than three to four weeks, see your physician because you may have a serious injury.

Achilles Tendonitis

The Achilles tendon is the cord that connects the calf muscles to the heel. Achilles tendon injuries occur particularly among people in poor physical condition. People over thirty years of age are also susceptible because the tensile strength (the amount of stress the tendon can bear without tearing) of their tendon lessens. Injuries to this tendon are common in start-and-stop sports such as tennis, racquetball, and basket-ball. Sprinting, jumping, and jogging, particularly jogging up hills, may also result in Achilles tendonitis. The injury ranges in severity from mild irritation to a complete severance of the tendon. If you felt a sudden sharp pain in your heel cord, you may have torn your Achilles tendon. This condition is serious and you should seek medical attention for it. However, you can deal with lesser injuries to the Achilles tendon yourself.

Achilles tendon problems don't seem to be related to running surface or body weight. Your running shoes, however, may be causing the problem. Wearing your flat tennis shoes is a sure invitation to this type of injury. If you want to run, be sure to buy shoes with a slight heel elevation. Most top quality jogging shoes have this feature.

The following is treatment for Achilles tendonitis:

●Ice massage the area or apply an ice pack with an elastic bandage for compression.

●Rest from your sport. Again swimming is a good conditioning alternative. The stationary bicycle may aggravate your injury—however, try it and see.

●Stretching your Achilles tendon will help you recover more rapidly. At first stretch by moving your foot slowly through its complete range of motion. You can do this lying down. Try to point your toes toward your shins, feeling a stretch in your heel cord. Next, get a towel or other long piece of cloth. Place the middle of the length of cloth around the ball of your foot. Pull back gently with the two ends until you feel a stretch. Hold the stretch for one minute, relax, then repeat this procedure five to ten times in a row and many times during the day. Stretch your Achilles tendon gently and statically. After some of the pain has dissipated, you can do the Achilles tendon stretching exercise on page 65.

•You can construct a slant board that will effectively stretch your heel cord. Build a ramp slanted at 45 degrees that's wide enough to stand on with both feet. Stand on the slant board and lean forward. You will feel a stretch in your heel cords. Hold the position for ten to thirty seconds at a time.

•When returning to your regular activities, begin by walking. Initially, avoid activities that involve rapid changes in direction and climbing up hills or stairs.

•Put a heel lift in your sports shoes. You can get these in a drug store that carries accessories for the feet. Re-examine the type of shoes you've been wearing. Sometimes a change in running shoes will make all the difference in the world.

•If the condition is particularly painful and seems to linger for many weeks, see a physician. You may have an anatomic abnormality in your foot that could be helped with an orthotic or your Achilles tendon may be torn.

•Taping the Achilles tendon may provide support during activity and prevent the tendon from stretching too far.

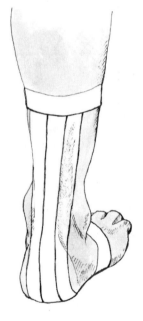

1. Place one anchor strip about three to four inches above the ankle joint and another just behind the ball of your foot.
2. Tear three strips of tape that are long enough to go over your heel from one anchor strip to the other.
3. With your foot in a neutral, unstretched position, overlap the three strips over your Achilles tendon, over your heel, and underneath your foot.
4. Place two locking strips over the anchor strips to hold the tape in place.

Achilles tendon pain can last many months if the injury is not taken care of properly. To prevent and treat Achilles tendonitis, it's particularly important to warm up properly before you run or play your sports. You should always do Achilles tendon stretching exercises prior to other exercises. With proper warm up and shoes, and gradual conditioning, you may be able to prevent this problem.

Achilles tendon taping procedure

Osgood–Schlatter Disease

Osgood–Schlatter disease is really an overuse injury rather than a disease. It is encountered principally among teenagers and is characterized by pain, swelling, and tenderness in the area just below the knee cap where the patellar ligament connects to the boney growth on the center of the upper part of the tibia (the large bone in your lower leg). Osgood–Schlatter disease is caused by repeated small tears at the point where the ligament connects to the bone. The condition occurs in girls between the ages of eight and thirteen and in boys between ten and fifteen. Boys are affected about three times more often than girls. Activities such as kneeling, direct contact with objects, running, and climbing may result in pain. I'm pointing out this problem because it does occur among young teenagers from time to time. With rest and restriction from activities, Osgood–Schlatter may clear up pretty quickly but probably not completely until growth ceases. You should see your physician if you suspect this problem.

Injuries to the Groin and Thigh Muscles

Injuries to the groin and thigh muscles are prevalent in sports requiring rapid movements and sudden changes in direction. Specific conditioning for this type of sport is essential to the prevention of injury to the large muscles of the thigh. Many people think that because they jog three to four miles a day they are physically prepared for basketball, tennis, skiing, or racquetball. Running will greatly enhance your conditioning, but to prevent injuries in these sports, you also must prepare yourself for fast movement.

Conditioning for sports requiring rapid movements should begin with jogging. After you are in fairly good shape, you can start sprint workouts. These should start with high speed runs on a 440 yard track. Sprint the straight-a-ways and walk the turns. Gradually decrease the distance of your sprints to fifty yards and less. When you feel comfortable with your straight sprint workouts, begin fast running in a zigzag pattern. Try to develop the ability to rapidly change directions while running full speed. Alternate this type of workout with runs up and down hills and on uneven terrain. In this way you will prepare your thigh and groin muscles for the high speed lateral movements required in many sports.

Groin Injuries

The groin is the area between the thigh and the stomach muscles. Few people have strong groin muscles and so this area is predisposed to injury. You can use the same exercises both to prevent injury and to rehabilitate groin muscles. The procedure for dealing with groin strains is similar to that for other muscle injuries.

- Periodically ice massage the injured area for several days.
- Rest the area for two to three days. When you return to activity, begin by walking and jogging. Gradually include running with changes of direction.
- Running in the shallow end of a swimming pool will aid in your rehabilitation.
- Gradually increase the muscle flexibility of the area with groin stretching exercises:

GROIN STRETCHER #1 Start in a seated position with heels together and close to the buttocks, knees apart. Push down on your knees until you feel a stretch in your groin. Hold the position for ten seconds. Relax, then repeat.

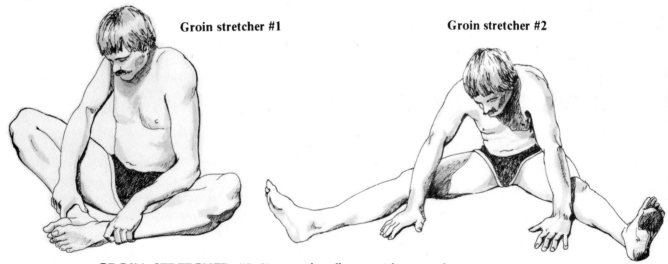

Groin stretcher #1   Groin stretcher #2

GROIN STRETCHER #2 Sit on the floor with your legs spread apart as wide as possible. Place your hands in front of you as far as possible until you feel a stretch in your groin and lower back.

GROIN STRETCHER #3 In a standing position, place one foot forward and one foot back, with legs spread well apart. Bend the forward knee and lean forward until you feel a stretch in the groin area of the leg that's in back. Switch legs and repeat.

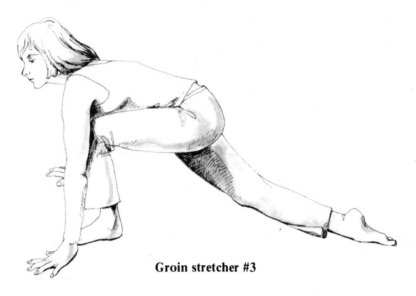

Groin stretcher #3

•You should attempt to strengthen your groin muscles after an injury. A good exercise is to have someone hold your legs about two feet apart. Attempt to pull your legs apart and then press them together as your partner provides resistance. You can also put two pillows between your knees and push your legs together.

Hamstring Injuries

Your hamstring muscles are located on the back of your upper legs. Hamstring injuries range in severity from microscopic tears to complete rupture. Ninety percent of these injuries occur where the muscle and tendon join on the outside portion of the hamstring (the muscle–tendon junction of the biceps femous muscle). In running, hamstring injuries occur during the foot-strike, the period when your foot hits the ground stopping the forward action of your leg. There is a lot of stress on these muscles at this time—particularly if your upper body is bent over (such as when you're bending over at the finish line of a sprint race). Many people who suffer hamstring injury have a strength imbalance between the muscles in the front (the quadriceps) and the rear of the thighs. Muscle imbalances result from doing a lot of quadriceps exercises such as stair climbing, hill running, sprinting, and knee bends without also doing strength exercises for the hamstrings. Generally, if your hamstrings are not at least 60 percent as strong as the muscles in the front of your thighs, you are risking an injury.

Your leg muscles are extremely powerful. When you run you must have cooperation between your hamstrings and quadriceps. When your quadriceps are working, your hamstrings must relax, and vice versa. When there is too large a strength difference between your quadriceps and hamstrings, your leg muscles don't cooperate the way they should and a muscle injury may result.

Treatment is similar to that of other muscle injuries:

● Ice massage the area intermittently until the symptoms disappear. Rest the area for two to three days. Wrap your thigh with an elastic bandage to provide compression. Try to elevate the leg.

● Begin rehabilitation with hamstring stretching exercises. These should be done very gradually. Hamstring pulls can sometimes be very serious and may take some time to heal. If not treated properly and conservatively, there is great danger of recurrence of the injury.

HAMSTRING STRETCHING EXERCISE #1 From a seated position on the floor with your legs stretched out in front of you, attempt to reach toward your toes until you feel a stretch in your hamstrings. Hold this position statically for ten seconds, relax, and then repeat. You can vary this exercise by placing your legs apart slightly and stretching.

Hamstring stretching exercise #1

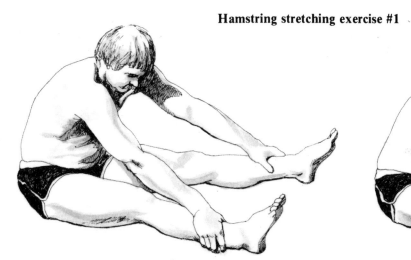

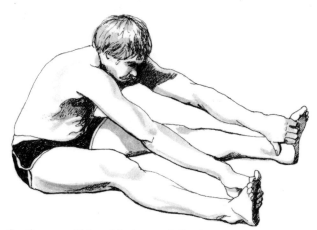

Reach as far as you can and hold the stretch.   **In time you'll be able to reach further.**

HAMSTRING STRETCHING EXERCISE #2 From a standing position, bend at the waist and let your arms hang down in front of you. Continue to bend until you feel a pulling in your hamstrings. Hold the stretch for ten seconds, relax, and then repeat. When returning to standing position after stretching, bend your knees—it's easier on your back.

Hamstring stretching exercise #2

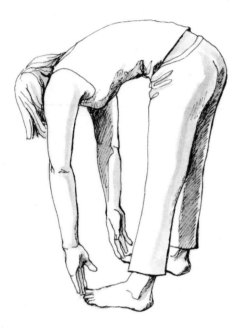

Let your arms hang and bend until you feel a stretch in your hamstrings.

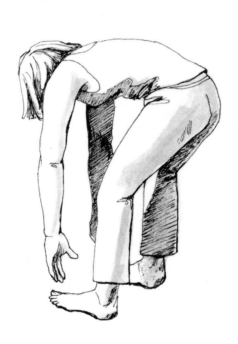

Bend your knees as you straighten up.

HAMSTRING STRETCHING EXERCISE #3 This exercise is sometimes called the hurdler stretch. For this exercise, assume a hurdler position, with one leg stretched straight in front and the other leg bent under your upper body. Move forward over your straightened leg until you feel a stretch in your hamstrings. Alternate legs and repeat the exercise.

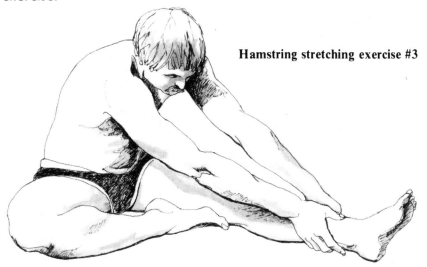

Hamstring stretching exercise #3

•Begin strengthening your hamstring three to four days following the injury:

HAMSTRING STRENGTH EXERCISE #1 From a standing or sitting position, contract your hamstring muscles, hold for ten seconds, relax, then repeat.

HAMSTRING STRENGTH EXERCISE #2 Lie on the floor on your stomach with your legs straight. Have someone provide resistance as you try to move your lower legs to a 90° angle with the floor.

HAMSTRING STRENGTH EXERCISE #3 Probably the best strength exercises for these muscles are the hamstring machines available at gymnasiums. Some sports medicine clinics have Orthotrons that allow you to train your hamstrings at high speed. If you have a serious hamstring injury, you should try to gain access to one of these machines to get maximum rehabilitation.

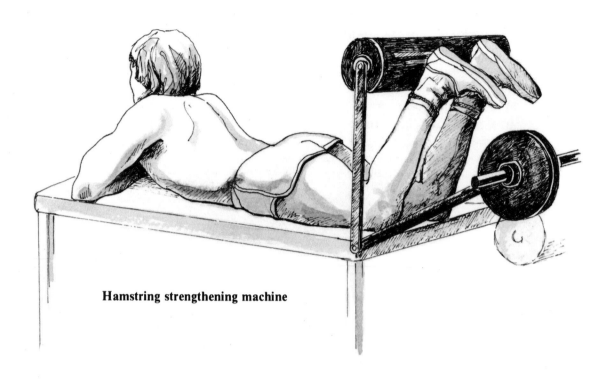

Hamstring strengthening machine

•As you try to return to your sport, increase the intensity of exercise gradually. Try to support your hamstrings with overlapping strips of athletic tape wrapped around your thigh. Dr. Donald Cooper, the team physician at Oklahoma State University, recommends wearing a woman's knee length panty girdle to support your injured hamstrings. Another alternative is to construct a neoprene sleeve from material available at a scuba diving shop.

Knee Pain

The knee is one of the most complicated and vulnerable joints in your body. Of all the people I know who have participated in sports for many years, few have escaped without at least some type of knee injury. The knee joint has a relatively unstable structure and is dependent upon muscles and ligaments for most of its support. Most people, particularly in the United States, do little to strengthen their legs. Weak and unfit leg muscles invite injury. Even weekend games of backyard volleyball, tennis, or skiing may make demands on your knee joints that they're not capable of coping with.

Knee injuries are often serious and often require treatment by an orthopedic specialist. Delay in seeking help from a specialist may result in damage that can be permanent, therefore self-help is not always the best path. Surgery is essential for certain ligament injuries. If it is delayed many debilitating conditions can occur. Your knee may degenerate because of too much looseness in the joint. You could develop traumatic arthritis that may affect you for the rest of your life. When you injure your knees, you should rely on the advice of a specialist. By following proper medical advice and by rehabilitation, you can minimize the effect of knee injuries on your sports participation and performance.

A wide variety of knee injuries fall into two basic categories:

- Traumatic
- Overuse

Traumatic knee injuries usually occur from a blow to the knee, forces directed to the sides of the knee, twisting of the knee, or hyperextension of the knee. Hyperextension occurs when the knee is forced backwards when it's already in a locked position.

One of the worst skiing injuries I ever had was falling on my knee in an icy parking lot. Blows to the knees are painful and can happen in almost any sport. Your knee has little padding, so it's particularly susceptible to this type of injury. You can protect yourself by wearing knee pads that can be purchased at any sports store for a few dollars. They may be valuable in sports such as volleyball, basketball, or skiing if you are susceptible to falling or getting hit.

A knee injury caused by a blow usually clears up in less than a week. Injury management initially includes the old first line of defense: ice, compression, and rest. Be sure not to use any heat while any swelling is present. Try to stay off your knee for a day or so. Try to move your knee through its normal range of motion and continue with ice massage during rehabilitation. If there's a lot of swelling or you're having too much pain, call your physician. This type of injury makes you susceptible to bursitis which may require additional rest and perhaps anti-inflammatory medication available from your doctor.

Knee sprains resulting from twisting or side forces directed toward the joint are sometimes difficult to deal with and are usually extremely frustrating. These injuries sometimes result in an unstable knee joint that can make you feel old before your time. Early surgery for completely torn ligaments is considered by orthopedics to be mandatory. The unstable knee joint must be dealt with and compensated for by muscle training or surgical reconstruction. Obviously, these alternatives call for the advice of an orthopedic specialist.

Treatment for a knee injury should include the following:

●After the injury, ice the knee. Wrap it with an elastic bandage and elevate it.

●Rest it. Use a pair of crutches to help you get around. Forget about the pro football player who gets a pain killer injected into his knee and returns to the game. Playing another set of tennis or running an extra couple of miles will make your injury worse.

●Have your injury evaluated by a physician within the first few days of the injury.

●Work to rehabilitate your knee as much as possible. These injuries take a long time to heal, and a weakened knee is easily reinjured. Your rehabilitation should include many types of exercise to prepare you for a variety of stresses.

●Perform knee strengthening exercises. You can increase the effectiveness of your knee strengthening exercises by applying ice massage for eight to ten minutes before and after your exercise session.

QUADRICEPS SETTING EXERCISE Tense the muscles in the front of your thigh. Hold the contraction for about ten seconds. Repeat this many times throughout the day. This exercise is especially good during the early stages of rehabilitation. It will keep your thigh muscles from atrophying (getting smaller) and, at the same time, not place too much strain on your injured joint.

LEG LIFTS WITH QUADRICEPS SETTING This exercise can be done as soon as you can tolerate it. Lie on your back with your legs straight. Then lift your injured leg to a 45 degree angle. Hold the position. As you get stronger, you can increase the resistance by using a weighted boot or sandbag, or you could have someone hold your leg.

KNEE EXTENSION AND FLEXION EXERCISES These should be started after you can do the leg lifts easily, when most of your range of motion is restored.

To perform knee extensions, sit at the edge of a table with knees bent at a 90 degree angle. Attach

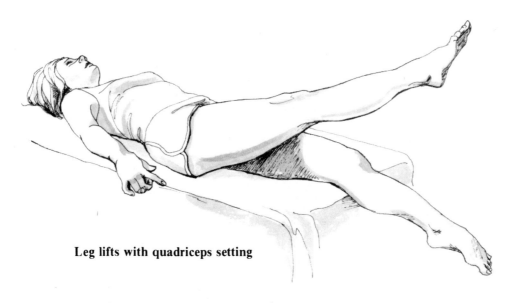

Leg lifts with quadriceps setting

weighted boots or sandbags to your shoes. Keeping your thighs on the table, straighten (extend) your leg. Knee flexion exercises can also be done with weighted boots. Lie face down on the floor or on a table with your leg straight. Keeping your thigh down, bend your leg.

Although you can use a weighted boot for these exercises, they are most effectively done with knee machines available at almost any health club. Isokinetic knee machines such as the Orthotron or Cybex (described in Chapter 3) are probably the ideal devices on which to do these exercises. They are available at sports medicine centers. If you decide to use weighted boots, be very careful. The weight of the boot and your leg hanging over the edge of a table may further injure your knee.

STAIR CLIMBING For some people, stair climbing is a good knee strengthening exercise. Start by walking up flights of stairs. Later you can run up. Stair climbing may be inappropriate if you have a condition called chondromalacia, sometimes called "runner's knee." In this condition you have a softening and roughening of the cartilage underneath your kneecap. Stair climbing and other exercises can aggravate chondromalacia. An orthopedic specialist can give you advice about the exercises that are best for you.

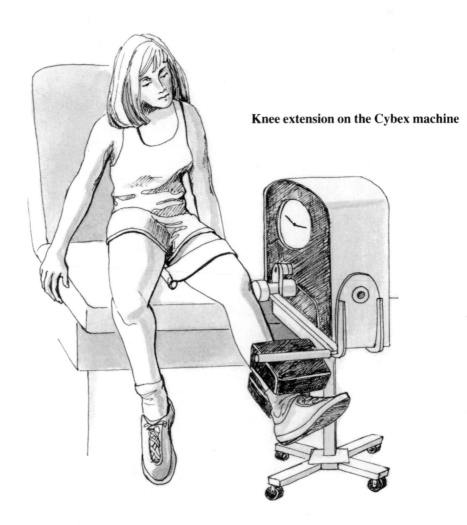

Knee extension on the Cybex machine

LEG PRESSES These are done on equipment available at a gymnasium and should be included as the strength of your knee improves. This exercise involves sitting on the seat of the leg press machine and pushing against a weighted lever using your feet and legs.

HEEL RAISES You should begin this exercise as soon as you can tolerate the movement. Begin by simply raising your heels and going up on your toes. As you get stronger, put a barbell on your back while doing the exercise to provide added resistance. Most gymnasiums have special heel raising machines.

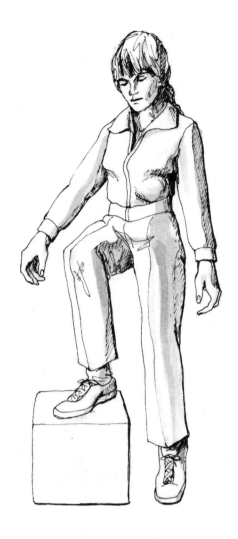

Bench stepping

BENCH STEPPING This is a good exercise if you don't have access to any equipment. Step up on a bench or stool. Your body weight serves as the resistance. To make the exercise more difficult, raise the height of the bench or put a barbell on your back to provide increased resistance.

● As the strength returns to your leg, you should attempt to regain normal function. Begin by walking long distances. As soon as you can walk three miles in less than forty-five minutes, you can begin jogging in a straight line. Be sure to run on a good surface such as a running track. A grass field or roadside may contain rocks or holes that may place additional strain on your knee if you encounter them. As your knee improves further, run large figure-eight patterns. With time, cut down the size of your figure eights until you are constantly and rapidly changing directions.

●Try to improve the endurance of your injured leg. Bicycling is an excellent way to do this. This type of exercise also contributes to your leg strength. Other endurance exercises include jogging and running in the shallow end of the pool, and leg kicks in the pool while holding onto the side. Water exercises are valuable because they allow you to exercise your leg muscles without putting too much weight on your injured joint.

●Exercise both the injured and uninjured leg. You actually increase the strength of your injured leg when you exercise the uninjured one. This is due to a phenomenon called cross-education. When you exercise your uninjured leg, signals are sent to your injured leg from your nervous system causing the injured leg to gain strength.

●Taping the knee is of little value. Because of the size and range of motion of the knee joint, the reinforcement capability of a knee taping is lost in a matter of minutes. Many medical experts recommend the Lenox-Hill brace. This brace increases stability but is uncomfortable and restricts movement. Ideally, you should depend upon the strength of your muscles to support your knee joint. If your knee is too weak to play tennis or volleyball, then it needs further rehabilitation before you return to play. Tape and most braces give you a false sense of security when you have a knee injury. There is no substitute for strong leg muscles.

●Motivation is extremely important when you're dealing with knee injuries. This disability can be extremely frustrating. You have to work very hard, consistently, over a long period of time. So, hang in there!

"Runner's Knee"

The term "runner's knee" has been used to describe a wide variety of knee pains that can be caused by several different factors. Because the diagnosis is nonspecific, there is no one treatment. The basic problem can range from tendonitis to chondromalacia.

Chondromalacia is a softening and roughening of the undersurface of the kneecap. It is believed to be caused by repeated traumatic injuries such as dislocations of the kneecap or by anatomic conditions that cause the kneecap to ride in an abnormal plane. If you can feel your knee grinding when you move it or if it's sometimes stiff or swollen, you may have developed chondromalacia. A sure sign of this condition is if you feel pain directly under the kneecap. Some people seem to be more prone to this condition than others. People involved in sports such as hiking or climbing, water or snow skiing, cycling, or running seem particularly susceptible to the problem.

Many chronic cases of runner's knee have been cleared up when the person runs on the outside of the foot. This can be accomplished through the use of orthotics or arch supports. Again, it's best to see a specialist if you have this problem—foot supports can help some types of knee pain but have no effects on others.

"Runner's knee" syndromes can be very difficult to deal with. The resulting knee pain can cause the strength and size of your knee to deteriorate because of the tendency to favor and protect the leg. This muscle weakness makes the joint more susceptible to sprains. Maintaining strength is essential, but you must follow some important principles.

● Avoid exercises that create pressure on your kneecap. Exercises that cause your knees to bend more than 90° will make the condition worse. Exercises and sports that may create problems include cycling, stair running, climbing, snow and water skiing, and knee extension exercises using weights.

● The best strength exercises for chondromalacia are done with isokinetic knee machines such as the Orthotron or Cybex. These machines, which allow you to exercise at high speeds, place less stress on the knee joint. High speed exercise has the advantage of developing strength without building up a lot of torque (force) in the knee joint. Straight-knee leg lifts with or without weights are good ways to build strength without further injuring the knee joint. Lie on your back on the floor—keeping your knee locked, raise your leg until it has reached a 45° angle. Hold the position for ten seconds, then relax.

● Tight quadriceps aggravate chondromalacia. You should be able to touch your heels to your buttocks easily. If you can't, you're too tight. The shin stretch exercise, page 65, should help to stretch your quadriceps.

Chondromalacia can be a difficult problem to deal with. You may have to resort to surgery to improve the condition.

Ankle Injuries

Sprained ankles can be particularly debilitating to your sports participation because there is a tendency to underrate them. "It's only a sprain" is an expression I've heard many times. On the other hand, "a sprained ankle is worse than a broken bone," is also a common belief. If you take proper care of an ankle injury, it needn't be a chronic problem. Generally, if full function to your ankle is not restored by ten minutes after an ankle injury, you should see a doctor. Early treatment of ankle injuries is essential if you are to avoid permanent problems.

Ankle sprains range in severity from mild, accompanied by swelling and pain but little injury to supporting ligaments; to moderate, with some injury to supporting ligaments; to severe, with complete tearing of ligaments. In some cases surgery is required to correct joint laxness and instability. In most cases, however, nonsurgical rehabilitation is the usual procedure. This rehabilitation process is extremely important since an ankle that's not fully recovered is easily subjected to further injury. I've seen many people give up tennis or basketball because of fear of ankle sprains when proper rehabilitation could have kept them on the court.

Lateral ankle sprains, those occurring on the outside part of the leg, account for about 85 percent of ankle injuries. Although the ankle is structurally more secure than the knee, the supportive musculature is weaker. Ankle sprains are prevalent in sports requiring rapid changes in direction such as basketball, tennis, and racquetball. Sports like gymnastics in which you might land off balance may also cause problems. Running on irregular surfaces, encountering gopher holes, rocks, and other such obstacles, may also cause you to sprain an ankle. Many shoe companies manufacture jogging shoes with flared heels that may help prevent this type of injury. Recent studies have shown that high-top tennis shoes help prevent ankle injuries in sports requiring rapid changes of direction.

The best way to prevent ankle sprains is to have strong and flexible foot, calf, and shin muscles. Some experts have suggested taping your ankles as a method of preventing sprains. This might be helpful if you have chronic problems, but it isn't necessary in a healthy individual. Taping can become a crutch and probably isn't that effective anyway. Tape on an ankle may loosen more than 75 percent during vigorous activity. It's better to develop a strong joint than to rely on tape.

Achilles tendon flexibility has been shown to be extremely important in preventing ankle sprains. Several professional sports teams have decreased the number of ankle injuries dramatically by emphasizing and practicing flexibility exercises on a regular basis.

Strive to regain stability in your ankle joint before you try to return to sports requiring rapid changes of direction. You should be able to run fast and change directions rapidly before you put your ankle to the test on the court. Again, the advice of an orthopedic specialist is important in helping you to make this decision. Returning to action too soon may result in a chronic condition.

The care of the sprained ankle is important. As with other muscle and joint injuries, the treatment should begin immediately.

● The immediate treatment for a sprained ankle is to apply an ice pack, wrap it with an elastic bandage, and elevate your leg. Gently point your foot downward and upward. These movements are called plantar and dorsiflexion. Avoid any twisting movement of the foot. Restrict your motion to an up-and-down motion in a plane that's in line with your leg. If your ankle is swollen or if the pain doesn't go away in ten minutes, you should see a doctor. A sprain to the inside of your ankle, or a medial sprain, often accompanies broken bones and should be x-rayed. A lateral ankle sprain, an injury to the outside of your ankle, can also involve broken bones.

● During the first few days after an ankle sprain, you should continue with ice, elevation, and compression. You can apply open ankle taping (see page 85) that will help support your ankle and aid in compression which reduces swelling. Open ankle taping allows for swelling yet provides reinforcement to the injured joint. You should work on range of motion exercises in the up-and-down plane only. Don't do any twisting motions with your foot until much of the swelling has subsided. You can do shin exercises that will help strengthen your ankle. Point your toes upward toward your shins and hold that position for ten seconds. Repeat this exercise periodically. You can maintain your cardiovascular fitness by riding a stationary bicycle or swimming. If you ride the bike, use your heels to pedal so that you avoid further ankle injury.

● As you begin to rehabilitate your injury, use a closed ankle taping to support the joint. Do the shin exercises with resistance. You can have someone hold your feet as you try to pull your toes toward your shins. You can also use an ankle rehabilitation machine such as the Orthotron to help you. You can begin the Achilles tendon stretching exercise (see page 65). Begin these very gently so that you don't reinjure the joint.

If most of the swelling has disappeared, you can start to do twisting movements with your foot to increase the range of motion. Don't do this until your ankle is starting to feel pretty good.

• It's important that you regain confidence in your injured ankle. As your ankle improves, try walking for extended periods. Walk up a hill that's relatively free of obstacles that could reinjure your ankle. Continue range of motion exercises, taping, and ice. Start doing some hopping in place and gradually integrate rope skipping in your program. Begin running in the shallow end of a swimming pool. Include short periods of jogging in your walking program. As your ankle recovers, increase the distance of your jogging.

• Try to restore your ability to move rapidly and change direction. Begin by sprinting in a straight line. Run backwards and sideways, using crossover steps, running to the side by placing one leg over the other as you move. Run in figure-eight patterns, gradually tightening the running course so that you are required to change direction rapidly.

• Continue to tape your ankle and apply ice during the total period of rehabilitation.

Closed Ankle Taping Procedure

Closed ankle taping is used to provide increased support during sports participation. Use open ankle taping, page 85, when there is a lot of swelling.

1. Apply an underwrap to your foot and leg to protect them from the tape. The underwrap could be thin foam rubber or a nylon stocking.
2. Apply an anchor strip about three inches above your ankle.
3. Apply two or three stirrup strips from the anchor strip on your leg, over the outside or lateral part of your ankle, under your foot, over the inside or medial part of your ankle, and back to the inside part of the anchor strip. Overlap the stirrup strips a little bit.
4. Apply a gauze or foam pad to the instep. Then apply cross strips—extend the cross strips so that they completely cover the top of the foot and shin.

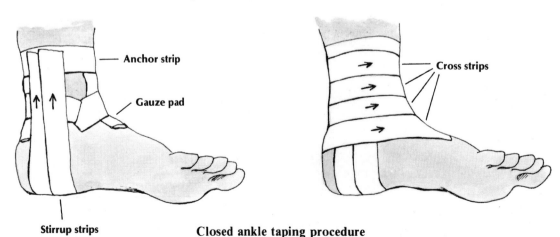

Closed ankle taping procedure

5. Apply a heel lock. This technique is used to keep the foot from moving from side to side and twisting. Begin the heel lock strip at the outside of the ankle. Tape across the instep and the inside part of the ankle, around the Achilles tendon, under the arch, and then back to the instep.

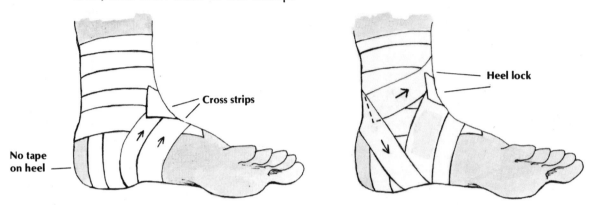

Tape applied directly to the skin will provide the most support. However, daily taping without an underwrap could lead to skin irritation. You should continue to tape your ankle for about three months following a severe ankle sprain. Don't, however, substitute tape support for the natural reinforcement you get from strong muscles and ligaments. Ligaments take a long time to heal. Their rehabilitation requires consistent hard work. Don't underestimate a sprained ankle. This type of injury can recur many times if it is not adequately cared for.

Open Ankle Taping Procedure

The open ankle taping technique is used when swelling is a problem. This is a good method to use during the first few days following an injury.

Follow the procedures for closed ankle taping but with these exceptions:

• When you apply the cross strips, leave a one-inch open area on the top of your foot and front of your shin.
• Wrap the taped ankle in an elastic bandage and you will receive support and compression.

Open ankle taping procedure

Foot Pain

Sore feet will stop you in your tracks. Running, skiing, tennis, racquetball, even swimming can cause foot injuries or foot pain. In skiing you can get sore feet from boots that don't fit right. In court sports such as tennis or racquetball you are susceptible to blisters. In swimming you may get sore feet from pushing off of the side of a swimming pool too many times. Unfortunately, the possibilities are endless.

Shoes

Let's start with running shoes. The athletics shoe industry does millions of dollars of business. We are deluged with a variety of information about running footwear—magazines publish shoe ratings, shoe companies bombard us with advertisements, and your running friends tell you about their favorite brand. Who are you to believe? The problem isn't that difficult because all of the big shoe companies manufacture fine products. Shoe design is a science, and these companies hire experts who design the shoes taking into consideration the biomechanics of running and the physical requirements of athletics. There are differences in running shoes, however. A shoe that may be good for your friend, or a model that has been rated number one by your favorite running magazine, may not be right for you.

When buying any shoe for sports, try to educate yourself about good and bad qualities of each brand. Get a variety of opinions. Take your time—a hasty decision may result in injury. First of all, get a pair of shoes that fit. Be sure to try the shoe on. Shoes made in Europe sometimes vary in fit from American shoes of the same size. Wear them in the store for a while to get the feel of them. Make sure the shoes provide good support—they should be firm but not tight. If they are too loose, you'll get blisters and foot irritations. The shoe should cushion the heel and the ball of your foot against shock. They should be flexible in the ball of the foot so that you can push off easily. The shoes should fit firmly in the heel—your feet should not ride up or you'll get blisters or you may irritate your Achilles tendon. You should be able to move your toes without pressure. If you have an unusual size foot, look around for shoes that can accommodate you properly. Some companies make shoes in varied widths and in extra long lengths. Buy shoes that are appropriate

What to look for in a running shoe

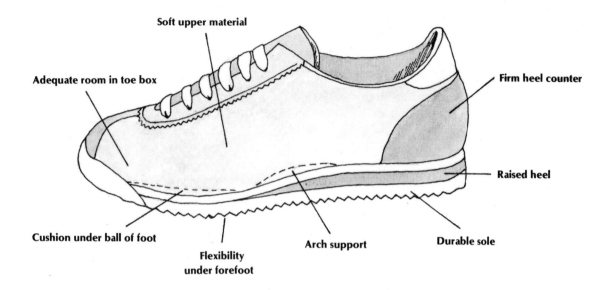

Soft upper material

Adequate room in toe box

Firm heel counter

Raised heel

Cushion under ball of foot

Flexibility under forefoot

Arch support

Durable sole

to your style of running. If you run on pavement, look for shoes designed to better absorb shock. If you run on irregular surfaces, get a shoe with a flared heel so that you have a little ankle stability. If you run in areas with a lot of mud or snow, make sure the soles provide good traction.

Beware of inexpensive imitations of the top running shoes. These are usually made of inferior materials that will not readily absorb shock and are not constructed with the same regard to the biomechanics of the foot. The thickness of the sole is not a good indication of a shoe's ability to absorb shock. A pair of those "five dollar wonders" may have thick soles, but can end up ruining your feet.

If you're playing court sports such as tennis, racquetball, basketball, or squash, it's best to buy shoes appropriate for these activities. Court shoes are made for rapid movements requiring changes of direction. If you play these games in your jogging shoes, you may easily develop blisters on the bottom of your feet or risk spraining your ankle. If you have trouble with your ankles, you might consider buying high-top tennis shoes. Studies have shown that high tops reduce the incidence of ankle sprains.

Ski boots give many people a lot of trouble because of their basic purpose—to maintain your foot in a rigid position. If your boots are loose, they may be very comfortable, but they will not provide the kind of support you need for skiing. The ski boot serves as an interface between your feet and legs, and your skis. You want to impart information from your body to your skis. If your boots are too loose, then your legs will do one thing and your skis another. Ski boots should fit snugly, but not tight. If they're too tight, your feet will get cold. Orthotics can, in some cases, aid in comfort and improve your skiing.

Shoes don't last forever. A worn shoe may cause you to become injured because your body is thrown out of balance. Shoes can be resoled by atheletic shoe specialists. In fact, there are companies that recondition your entire shoe at a price that's much less than a new pair. With the price of shoes continuing to escalate, reconditioning your old ones may be an attractive alternative.

Socks

The wrong socks can be a source of foot irritation. The best socks for running and tennis are made of cotton. Avoid socks that bind your toes or you'll get blisters and toenail irritations. In skiing and backpacking you might want to wear two pairs of socks: an ultrathin inner pair and a wool outer pair. Since two pairs of socks do much to reduce friction, the two-sock approach is also successful for runners.

Blisters on the ball of the foot can be a problem in sports like tennis and basketball. They are particularly prevalent during the first part of the season—those first few days out on the court. Harry Anderson, former football coach and currently teacher of an athletic injury course at San Jose State University, has a suggestion that works: apply petroleum jelly to the outside of your socks. This really cuts down on the friction and will reduce your blister problems.

Injuries to Your Arches

Your foot has two arches: one under the ball of your foot, the metatarsal arch, and another in the middle of your foot, the longitudinal arch. Many people develop pain in foot arches at one time or another. These may be sudden strains or they can be more subtle. You may wake up in the morning and have sore, stiff feet from overuse. The pain usually goes away after you walk around for a while.

Metatarsal arch strain is common among joggers. You can develop this condition if you run on hard surfaces, wear shoes that don't fit, or overtrain. The severity of this injury ranges from moderate to severe disability. Longitudinal arch strains, although in a different part of the foot, are similar in nature and call for similar treatment patterns. The care for these injuries should be conservative:

●Rest—an arch injury can easily become a chronic condition. Try to keep your weight off the ball of your foot for a few days. Keep your conditioning by swimming or bicycling (if you bicycle, pedal with your heels).

●Try changing your running shoes. Some people's feet can't tolerate certain types of shoes. A shoe that's perfectly adequate for running on grass may produce injury on the sidewalk.

●If you are overweight, lose a few pounds. Excess fat does lead to arch injuries. If you are more than fifteen or twenty pounds overweight, it's best that you restrict your endurance exercise to non-weight bearing activities such as bicycling or swimming. Walking may be appropriate because your feet aren't subjected to as much shock.

●Ice, and after two days, contrast heat and ice will help dissipate pain and assist you in doing foot exercises.

●Developing strong and flexible foot muscles is important. Do foot exercises such as picking up marbles with your toes or rolling up a towel with your feet. Try to contract and move as many muscles in your feet as possible. Curl your toes and twist your feet using all your foot muscles.

•Taping the arches can sometimes provide comfort and support.

Metatarsal Arch Taping
This procedure tapes the arch at the ball of the foot.

1. Cut three strips of tape long enough to go around your foot at the ball.
2. Cut an oblong ⅛-inch thick felt pad that will fit just behind the ball of your foot. Wrap the strips loosely around the pad, taking care not to constrict or compress the foot.

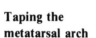

**Taping the
metatarsal arch**

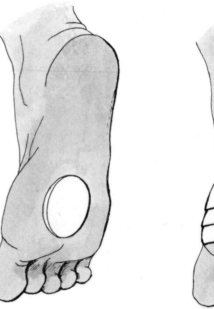
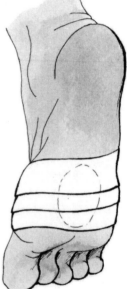

Longitudinal Arch Taping
This procedure tapes the large arch in the middle of the foot.

1. Cut three strips of tape long enough to fit around the middle of your foot.
2. Place a ¼-inch thick foam pad on your arch and wrap it with the tape strips.

•A podiatrist or foot specialist may be able to provide orthotic devices that can help support injured arches. The important thing is not to let this type of injury go too far. If conservative treatment doesn't do the trick, see a foot specialist with a knowledge of sports medicine.

Heel Pain

Heel bruises are common among runners due to the shock received from the constant pounding of jogging. Like other overuse injuries of the foot, heel bruises are difficult to get rid of and can become chronic conditions if not taken care of. The treatment for this injury should be gradual and often requires patience:

●Rest is crucial. You should try not to put much weight on your heel if you can help it. Use alternative means of exercise such as swimming to stay in condition.

●Ice therapy should be used during the first few days of disability.

●Examine your shoes. Heel bruises can be a problem with certain brands and can disappear when you change shoes.

●Put foam rubber heel cushions in your shoes. These can be purchased in any drug store.

●When you return to training, put plastic heel cups in your shoes. You can buy them at a sports store or a running specialty shop. The heel cup will help dissipate the shock of running.

Blisters and Calluses

Blisters and calluses can be a problem if you don't have shoes and socks that fit correctly. They may be inevitable if you overdo a sport such as tennis or racquetball. You need time to condition your feet properly to start-and-stop sports. If you push too hard during the early phases of your conditioning, you will feel like the bottoms of your feet are burning up.

Blisters are overuse injuries of the skin. Broken blisters should be cleaned with soap and water, and antiseptic. If the blister is in bubble form, penetrate the base with a sterilized needle to drain the fluid. Sterilize the needle with a match or over a flame. Cover the blister with an adhesive bandage or with a piece of moleskin, available at drug stores, to protect it from further injury. Blisters can easily become infected if not kept clean. If infection does occur, see your physician.

Calluses form on your feet from the irritation of shoes being too loose or too tight. Certain foot abnormalities can make you more susceptible to this problem. If this is the case, a foot specialist should evaluate you. Don't cut calluses with a razor. A pumice stone can be used to keep the size of a callus down. Rub the area with oil or lanolin to prevent the callus from cracking. Covering the callus with moleskin can lessen the effect of friction from your shoes. Placing an inner sole in your shoe may also help this condition.

Toenail Problems

Toenails can become embedded in the surrounding skin. An ingrown toenail can be extremely painful and make normal movements very difficult. There are two things you can do to prevent toenail problems: trim your toenails straight across and get shoes that are both the right width and the right length for you. If you get an ingrown toenail, you can attempt to relieve the problem by pushing some cotton under the nail where it's ingrown. If this doesn't help or if the problem recurs, you should consider seeing your doctor and having the ingrown side of your toenail removed.

Another condition encountered in sports is an accumulation of blood under the toenail. This can happen from playing in shoes that don't fit, running up hills, or from jamming your toes (such as when you kick an object too hard). If the condition doesn't cause you any pain, don't worry about it. Your toenails may look awful, but functionally there will be no problem. (You can always paint them.) During the first twenty-four hours after the blood accumulates, you can melt a hole in your nail with a hot paper clip and drain the blood. Heat the paper clip until it is red-hot with a match or over a flame. Be careful not to go in too deep. This procedure is painless and should help relieve much of the pain. Be sure to clean and bandage the area.

Athlete's Foot: There's a Fungus Among Us

Athlete's foot is a catchall term used to describe fungus infections. The condition is characterized by a rash and itching. You can prevent infection by regularly washing and drying your feet. After a bath, make sure you dry between your toes. Try to wear clean, dry socks, and use talcum or cornstarch in your shoes. If you develop athlete's foot, you can purchase athlete's foot medication at a drug store. Severe skin problems should be examined by a dermatologist.

Instant Replay

- Lower body injuries can be prevented by gradual conditioning.
- Proper leg strength and flexibility is critical in preventing leg injuries.
- Serious joint injuries should be evaluated by an orthopedic specialist. Joint laxity may cause deterioration that may lead to chronic pain.
- Good shoes are very important for injury prevention. You should buy a good quality shoe that fits you properly and is appropriate to your sport.

5.

INJURIES TO THE TRUNK AND HEAD

Jim was an unlikely candidate for early retirement from the police department due to severe back pain. He looked more like a participant in the Mr. America Contest than a backache invalid. He had large, powerful looking arms and shoulders, a small waist, and two large muscular bulges running up his back that resembled a pair of boa constrictors. Understandably, the civil service commissioners looked upon Jim's claim with a great deal of skepticism.

"I can find nothing structurally wrong with his back," declared the examining physician. "There are no ruptured discs or broken bones."

"Doctor, do you mean he may be faking his injury?" queried one of the commissioners.

"No, not necessarily," said the doctor. "I mean I can't find any evidence of injury to his back. He may indeed have severe back trouble; I just can't determine the cause."

The commissioners retired to another room to discuss the case. "Just another guy trying to get a permanent meal ticket from the City!" "Well, he's not going to get away with it! With arms like that, he should be unloading boxes at City Hall, not complaining about a sore back."

The commissioners re-entered the room and quickly denied Jim's request for disability.

Many very physically fit people like Jim have back trouble. In fact, about 80 percent of the population will have a back disorder at one time or another. Many times the causes are difficult to determine, but the pain is very real to the person with the backache. If you heed a few simple principles, you may be able to prevent back trouble.

The Causes of Trunk Injuries

A favorite topic of discussion among physical anthropologists is the many aches and pains caused by man's erect posture. Man's evolution as a standing animal is considered incomplete by many experts and thus human anatomy is sometimes poorly equipped for coping with the trauma and overuse experienced in sports and physical exercise. As with the athletic injuries already discussed, it's best to avoid back problems rather than treat them. There is no substitute for strong, flexible muscles and a solid, correct posture. A back brace is a poor alternative for a versatile anatomy that's ready for a variety of movements and physical stresses.

Your body is maintained in an erect posture by your spinal column, a collection of bones called vertebrae. The seven bones in your neck and upper back are called cervical vertebrae. The twelve vertebrae in the middle of your back are called thoracic, and the lower five vertebrae are called lumbar. The vertebrae are connected to two other bones, the sacrum and the coccyx (tail bone). The sacrum is supported by your pelvis. This total structure is constructed for two sometimes conflicting functions:

•To enable you to maintain an erect posture against the forces of gravity
•To allow you the flexibility and capacity for movement in this upright position

Your spinal column possesses a series of curves. If you could view the profile of the skeleton with x-ray eyes, you would see a convex curve in the upper part of the spine, a concave curve in the middle, and another convex curve in the lower. The proper balance of these curves is extremely important in preventing injury. A balanced spine requires very little muscular support. The mechanical structure of the vertebrae column and its supporting ligaments successfully maintain an erect posture. As soon as the body moves out of a balanced posture, your muscles must move in to support your body structure. If an imbalance is chronic, due to such factors as mechanically unsound body positions, your muscles will fatigue easily and you will be subject to trunk injury. These injuries can occur anywhere along the length of the spine from the neck to the lower back.

Trunk injuries are easier to understand if you know the basic structure of the vertebrae. The front of the vertebrae supports the weight of the body in the upright posture; the back of these bones guides the movements of the spine. In between the bones are shock absorbing structures called discs. Trunk pain can be caused by a variety of factors related to aberrations in the structure of your spine. Pain can also be caused by injury to trunk ligaments and muscles, injury or pressure on spinal nerves, and irritation in the joints of the various vertebrae themselves.

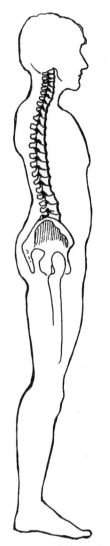

The curves of the spine

Lower Back Pain

Lower back problems are common among people involved in sports and exercise. Many of us have had the experience of overexercising only to get a sore back that evening or the next day. Extreme care must be taken in dealing with lower back pain in order to avoid a chronic condition. You must be sure to follow the basic first aid procedures, get the proper amount of rest, and make sure you fully rehabilitate and recondition your back.

The prevention of lower back injury is complicated because other areas of the body are involved in addition to the muscles and ligaments of the lower back. Prevention of lower back pain includes maintaining or developing the following:

- Strong and flexible back muscles
- Strong abdominal muscles
- Good flexibility in the hamstrings, hip flexors, and Achilles tendon
- Good posture
- Good sports techniques and body mechanics
- Adequate strength in the legs and buttocks

All of these factors are interrelated and interdependent. If you haven't got back problems now, you should be aware of these factors as preventative measures. If you do have backache, then you should work very hard and consistently to correct deficiencies in as many of these areas as possible.

Sports and exercise often require you to move quickly and forcefully. If you have a sound structure and good body mechanics, then there is little risk of injury. Whenever you move from a static standing position, your muscles are called upon to maintain balance and support the new position. Bending down, for example, requires a reversal in the convex curve of your lower spine and a simultaneous tilting of your pelvis. Movements like this present no problem if you have the necessary muscle strength and flexibility and neuromuscular coordination. However, if you don't, you may be susceptible to back pain and injury.

With good posture and good technique, you can prevent back pain. When the body is out of balance, the muscles must increase their assistance. As they fatigue there is danger of straining the ligament support of the spine, thus creating back injury and pain. The most important factor in balancing the spinal curves is the relationship between the pelvis and the vertebrae in the lower back. If poor posture and weak, inflexible muscles allow the curvature of the lower back to increase to a sway back position then back pain will almost always ensue. During exercise the relationship of the pelvis to the spine is also critical. If the pelvis is unable to tilt forward as you bend over, you can easily injure your back.

Correct sports techniques are also important in preventing back problems. If your movements are jerky and unpredictable, you can easily exceed the capacity of your back structure and become injured. You should be aware of proper lifting techniques and methods of controlling your center of gravity so that the large, strong muscles of your body, rather than the muscles of your back, are controlling your movements. (Proper lifting techniques are described on page 102.)

Posture and Backache

As a boy I had a teacher who was adamant about good posture. "Stand up straight. Tom," she would say. "Be proud of your height. Don't slouch in your chair. Educated people don't slouch." The teacher was a classic Victorian school marm who resembled Miss Grundy of the "Archie" comic strip. For years I thought her ideas on posture were a throwback to her quaint and genteel upbringing. It never occurred to me at the time that posture and body mechanics are the cornerstones of a healthy back.

With good posture, you should be able to remain standing or seated for a reasonably long period of time comfortably and with little effort. Your bones and their ligamentous attachments should be aligned so that little muscular exertion is required to maintain a particular body position. However, when you assume an inefficient body posture, your muscles are called upon to assist. They can easily fatigue and stress the joints and ligaments of your spine that are so critical for maintaining painless postures.

Although there are some bad posture characteristics that are due to structural abnormalities and genetics, most problems of this nature are due to bad habits developed over the years.

There are certain postures that are characteristic of the way you feel psychologically. The athlete, after losing an important game, is often slumped and dejected. His head is bowed forward and he may walk with a slow shuffle. This is the classic "agony of defeat" posture. Many people with negative attitudes about themselves may also assume this type of drooped stance on a chronic basis. These postures quickly fatigue and stress the supportive structures of your back.

As you can see, dealing with back pain is not simply a matter of doing a few exercises fifteen minutes a day. A chronically angry or impulsive person may be setting the stage for back pain by assuming tense postures, creating tight muscles, and performing movements that are abrupt and potentially damaging to the spine and its supporting structure. A few exercises will not make up for twenty-four hours of bad posture or a tense and anxiety-ridden lifestyle. Dealing with posture related back pain, then, is a matter of:

- Correcting bad posture habits
- Strengthening muscles and developing flexibility in areas necessary for good posture
- Reducing anxiety and developing a positive attitude about yourself

The angle between your pelvis and lower spine is the most important factor in posture-related back pain. Body positions that allow your pelvis to tilt forward and cause your back to arch should be avoided. You can do a lot to correct many painful back problems by maintaining good posture in three common body positions: lying, standing, and sitting.

When you sleep, try to avoid any position that causes your back to arch. Sleep on a bed firm enough to provide the necessary support to your spine. A soft bed that sags in the middle may cause you to wake up every morning with a backache. If you start the day with back pain, your sleeping habits or your bed may be part of the problem. Water beds have become relatively popular in recent years and have been advocated as good for the prevention of backache. Under ideal circumstances they do provide even support of your body weight. However, if the beds are not filled with the correct amount of water or you sleep on the edge of the "mattress," you may end up in a bad sleeping position. I had a water bed for years. Usually it worked out very well, but if I slept too near the edge of the bed, I would end up sleeping in the space between the mattress and the frame. That particular position wasn't too good for my back.

If you sleep on your back, you should prop up your legs with pillows or spare blankets so that you flatten your lower spine. Various companies sell beds that mechanically raise the knees. If you have back trouble and have the money, you might consider investing in one. Avoid sleeping on your stomach since this position makes your back arch. Probably the best sleeping position is on your side with your knees bent. This sleeping posture puts you in a good anatomical position.

Prop your legs up with pillows if you sleep on your back.

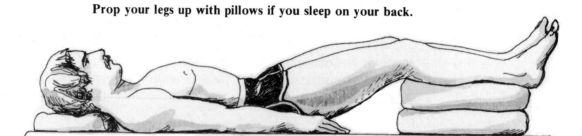

If you are standing on your feet for a long time, you should take precautions to protect your back. The powerful muscle group ilio-psoas is responsible for hip flexion (moving your thigh toward your trunk). When you're in a standing position, this muscle group tends to tilt your pelvis forward, causing your lower back to arch. By propping your foot on a box, you can straighten your lower back and place less strain on your postural muscles. In the past, saloons had a railing about three or four inches from the floor. Its purpose was to provide back support for the customers. Few modern bars or discos provide this anymore. They are producing a generation of inebriated people with backache.

Many people have jobs that require them to sit for long periods during the day; "secretary spread" is only one of the results. If you work at a desk or drive a car or truck for long periods, you should take great care to maintain a good seated posture. Your chair should allow your lower back to be relatively straight. The seat and back should be firm and be at a height that allows your knees to bend at a 90 degree angle and your feet to rest on the floor. If the chair is too low, the resulting angle between your torso and thighs can cause strain and back fatigue. If the chair is too high, it will force you to bend over and cause back fatigue. Try to sit without crossing your legs.

A prerequisite of good posture is adequate muscle strength and flexibility. Specific exercises to help you develop these things begin on page 103. Generally, you should develop strong, flexible back muscles, strong stomach and leg muscles, and flexible hip and hamstring muscles. Good back exercises are directed at developing an ideal angle between your spine and pelvis. If you have back trouble, you should avoid exercises that cause you to arch your back (back hyperextension exercises). Hyperextension exercises are great for strengthening the lower back for sports in the absence of backache. These are common exercises among athletes and are even incorporated into commercial weight training machines, such as the Universal Gym.

Relaxation and reduction of anxiety are extremely important for reducing back pain. Muscle spasms—painful uncontrolled muscle contractions—accompany back injuries and are worse in the tense, anxious individual. If you are a so-called Type A individual, the nervous excitable person, you might consider trying some of the popular techniques available today to combat the effects of stress. Two of the most popular methods are transcendental meditation (TM) and progressive relaxation. Although I think that some of the claims made by the proponents of TM are scientifically unsound, this technique has been shown to be effective for stress reduction in many people.

Body Mechanics and Your Back

As I mentioned earlier, part of the vulnerability of the back is due to its sometimes contradictory functions: postural support and trunk mobility. Improper lifting techniques or sudden stresses upon postural muscles can cause injuries that may result in ligament laxity in turn resulting in chronic back pain.

Your level of skill in a sport has a great deal to do with your susceptibility to injury. A skilled person knows how much force to exert and when to brace for a sudden jolt. A beginner may exert too much power and can severely overwhelm the muscles and supportive ligaments in the back. The beginners movements are often jerky and off-balance and these, too, increase the risk of an injury.

Many factors are involved in lower back pain. The problem may not be in the back at all. Many runners have found relief from back pain by consulting a foot doctor who corrected an existing difference in leg strength or structural abnormality in the foot. Muscle strength and flexibility in the legs and trunk are critical in maintaining the proper lower back curve. Tight hamstrings and weak abdominals create a swayback position in the body at rest; the force exerted during exercise increases the likelihood of straining these incorrectly positioned back muscles.

Poor lifting techniques are a common cause of many back injuries. In sports and exercise, it's easy to overwhelm back muscles if proper techniques are not observed. To lift properly:

• Keep the weight as close to your body as possible. The farther a weight is held from your body, the more strain there is on the back.

• Do most of the lifting with your legs. The large muscles of your thighs and buttocks are much stronger than your back muscles which are designed basically to help you maintain an erect posture. Keep your hips and buttocks tucked in.

• Don't bend at the waist with straight legs to pick something up. This action places tremendous strain on your back.

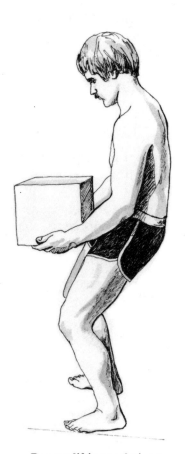

Proper lifting technique

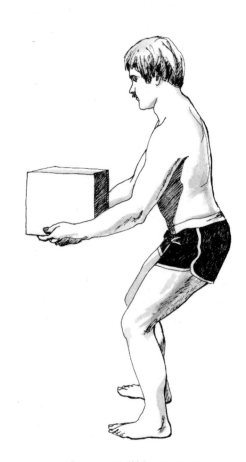

Improper lifting technique

Exercises for Your Back

These exercises can be used both in the prevention and treatment of back pain. They should be done gradually—start off easily and progressively increase the intensity. If your back hurts, you will get much more from the exercises if you get someone to apply ice massage before and after your workout. Ice will help reduce muscle spasms and make the exercises easier and less painful. Do these exercises two times every day. Exercises for the back include stomach exercises, hamstring flexibility exercises, hip flexibility exercises, thigh strengthening exercises, and Achilles tendon flexibility exercises, in addition to flexibility and strength exercises for the back itself.

KNEE LIFTS Lie on your back with your legs straight. Put both of your hands under your left knee—raise your left knee to your chest; keep the other leg straight. Hold the left knee to your chest for five seconds. Repeat this exercise with the other leg. Relax and repeat this series.

DOUBLE KNEE LIFTS Pull both knees to your chest while lying on your back. Hold this position for five seconds; relax, and repeat.

Double knee lifts

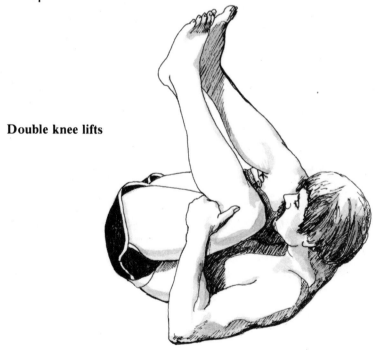

SUPER KNEE LIFTS This exercise is a continuation of the double knee lift. Lie down on your back and bring your knees to your chest. Brace yourself by putting your hands on the floor next to your hips. Next, extend your legs and roll onto your shoulders and attempt to touch the floor behind your head with your feet. Support your back with your hands. Hold this position for five seconds.

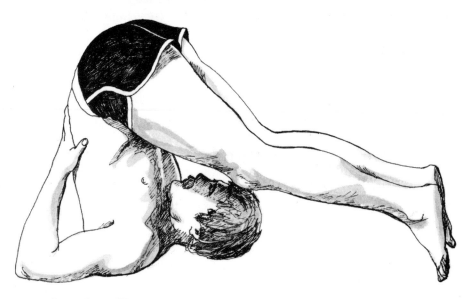

Super knee lifts

PELVIC TILTING This exercise helps you develop a good angle between your pelvis and your spine.

It's best to perform this exercise initially on a hard floor or carpet. Lie down on your back with your knees bent. Press your lower back to the floor and elevate your buttocks. You will feel the stretch along your lower back. Hold the position for five seconds at a time, relax, then repeat. Start off with a few repetitions, gradually increasing the frequency as your back gets stronger. After you become accustomed to realigning your pelvis and lower back, you can perform this exercise standing, kneeling, or sitting.

Pelvic tilting

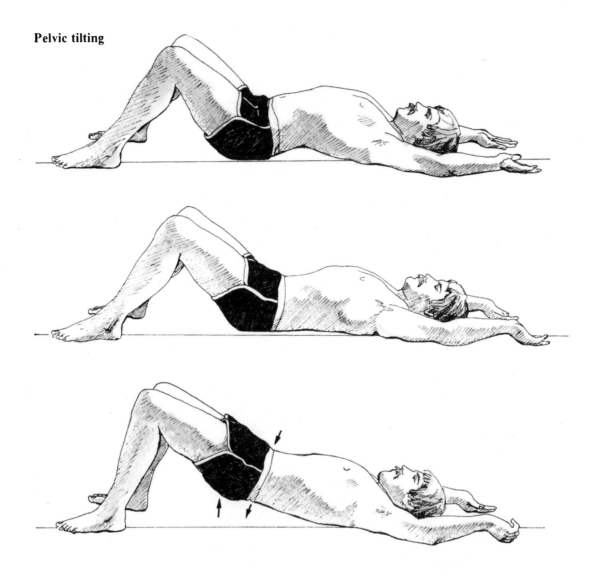

There is an alternate to this exercise that you can do in bed. Lie on your back with your knees bent, then contract your stomach and buttocks muscles while pressing down on your lower back.

HAMSTRING STRETCHING EXERCISES Hamstring flexibility is extremely important in the prevention and treatment of back pain. Do the hamstring stretches beginning on page 71. Remember, when you stretch your hamstrings, don't bounce—just hold the stretched position for ten seconds or so, then relax.

ACHILLES TENDON STRETCHING Ankle flexibility can also be related to back pain. (As you can see, back injury can be extremely complex.) Do the Achilles tendon exercise on page 65.

ABDOMINAL CURLS These are similar to sit-ups except you don't go all the way up. Abdominal curls are preferable to sit-ups during the early stages of back rehabilitation because less strain is placed on your spinal muscles. Lie on your back with knees bent. Curl your upper body about four inches from the floor, then bring it back down. Your lower back stays in contact with the floor during this exercise.

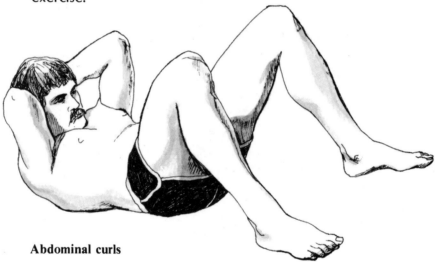

Abdominal curls

SIT-UPS Strong abdominal muscles are extremely important in preventing back pain. If your stomach muscles sag, your back will arch to compensate for the redistribution of weight. Sit-ups are the classic abdominal exercise.

For this exercise, lie on your back, bend your knees, and place your feet flat on the floor. Have someone hold your feet or hook them underneath a couch. This bent knee position will keep your lower back straight when you're lying on the floor. With your hands crossed over your chest, lift your trunk until your chest touches your thighs. As you develop stronger stomach muscles, do the exercise grasping your hands behind your head. You can also twist while doing the movement, touching your right elbow to your left knee and vice versa. Begin with two to ten repetitions of this exercise. As you become stronger, increase the amount (the world record for sit-ups is well over 10,000).

STOMACH TIGHTENERS This is an exercise you can do anywhere: at the office, in the garden, in your car, in your bed. All you have to do is tighten and hold in your stomach for ten seconds and relax. Repeat periodically during the day. You can increase the benefit of this exercise by simultaneously contracting your buttocks muscles.

HANDS AND KNEES EXERCISE Get down on your hands and knees. Hang your head down and curve your back upward while holding your stomach in. Relax and repeat.

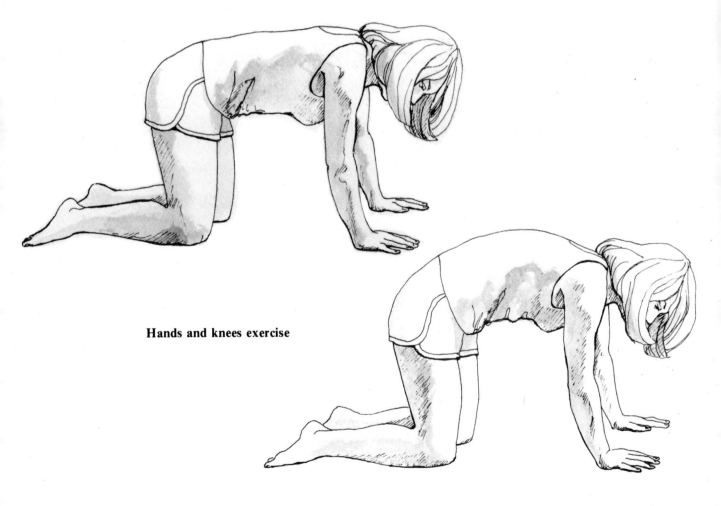

Hands and knees exercise

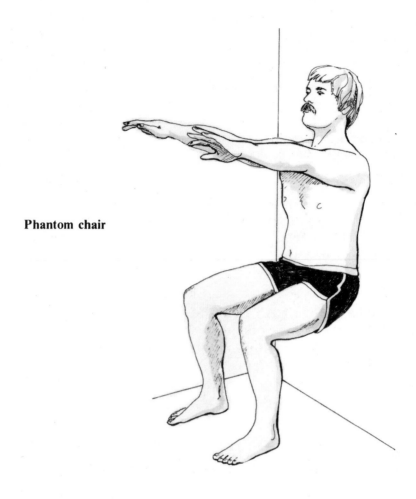

Phantom chair

PHANTOM CHAIR Brace your back against a wall or pole with your knees bent at a 90 degree angle. (You should be in a seated position—without a chair). Stay in this position for as long as you can.

HIP STRETCHERS Put your hands on the floor, bend one knee, and extend the other leg behind you. Push forward and downward on the bent knee. You should feel a stretch in your extended leg and your pelvis. Reverse the position of your legs and repeat.

Injuries to the Back

Bruises

Your back has a large surface area that makes it susceptible to bumps and bruises during exercise. They can occur in sports such as basketball, skiing, racquetball, or any activity where you could bang into another person or object. Bruises usually involve your back muscles rather than the vertebrae, which are pretty well protected. When you sustain a sudden trauma of this nature, you'll typically experience swelling, pain when you move, muscle spasms, stiffness, and restriction of movement. The treatment of back bruises is similar to treatment for bruises in other parts of your body.

●Massage the area with ice for ten minutes or apply an ice pack for thirty minutes as soon as possible after the injury. Repeat several times during the day and continue for two to three additional days.

●See a doctor if you suspect the bruise might be serious.

●Don't use aspirin for about a week after this injury—aspirin affects the blood's ability to clot and may make the injury worse.

●You can use heat after three days of ice treatment. A good technique is to alternate between ice and heat treatments. Appropriate heat treatments include a hot shower, hot whirlpool, hydrocollator packs, or hot water bottle (see page 50). If you take a hot bath, don't sit with your legs straightened. This position increases the curve of your lower back and may make your condition worse.

●Try to rest for the first day or so after the injury. You should include some range of motion exercise to prevent stiffness (see page 103).

●Consider taping a foam rubber pad over the area for protection if it seems appropriate.

●When you return to sports, apply ice massage immediately after exercise. This will minimize any internal bleeding that may occur if the bruise is not completely healed.

Strains and Sprains

Strains are injuries to the muscles and tendons in your back; sprains are injuries to your spinal ligaments. As with most athletic injuries, you should seek the advice of a physician if the injury is at all serious. An x-ray examination will determine whether there are broken bones. Back strains and sprains are caused by physical overexertion or violent stretching or contractions that overwhelm the structures of your back. These injuries can be severely debilitating and should be dealt with quickly and effectively. You can easily recognize the symptoms: muscle spasms, pain when you move, loss of strength and movement capacity, discoloration, and sometimes pain when you touch the area. You can distinguish between a strain and a sprain by isometrically contracting your lower back muscles against some immovable resistance—you will feel pain with a strain, but not a sprain.

The following is a treatment program for back sprains and strains.

- Use ice massage or an ice pack for the first few days. This therapy should begin immediately after the injury and be repeated as often as possible (once every one to two hours while you're awake) during the day.
- If you hurt your back, stop playing. You may feel as if you can keep going, but you'll feel a lot worse later if you do. A hurt back will stiffen up but you can keep this to a minimum if you rest after the injury.
- Lie down on a firm mattress on your back with your knees elevated.
- See a doctor if the pain is severe.
- After twenty-four to thirty-six hours you can begin gradual back flexibility and strength exercises, as pain permits. Remember, some pain is inevitable. You have to try to maintain range of motion in your back, but don't overdo it either.
- Swimming is often a good exercise when recovering from back sprains and strains providing you don't arch your back when you breathe. You can prevent arching by using a snorkel when you swim— this will allow you to breathe without hurting your back.
- You can begin running as the pain diminishes. Try to jog on soft surfaces at first. Ice the area after you exercise.
- Concentrate on good posture and body mechanics. Be careful to use proper lifting techniques.

Disc Injuries

Between your vertebrae are shock absorbing pads called discs. The discs are composed of a fibrous material filled with a gel-like substance. With years of wear and tear, your discs may lose some of their shock absorbant qualities and begin to degenerate. Physical fitness and muscle tone is extremely important for maintaining healthy discs. By adhering to good habits of posture and body mechanics and remaining physically fit, you are much less likely to have problems with these structures.

A rupture of a disc can put pressure on your sciatic nerve creating a condition called sciatica. Sciatica can cause referred pain anywhere along the path of the nerve ranging from your buttocks to your foot. If you feel a pain running down your leg when you cough or sneeze, you may have a disc problem. As with any serious problem concerning your health, consult your physician.

Back Braces

A back brace is not a substitute for strong muscles. The function of a back brace is to support the abdominal muscles and prevent the lower back from arching. Your doctor can prescribe a brace that will work for you if one is necessary. Many commercially available elastic braces are inadequate because they don't provide enough support. Many people use a large neoprene wrap as a brace for exercising and it is a technique recommended by many physicians. You can make one of these from material available at a scuba diving store. They tend to make you sweat so when you finish exercising, be sure to dry off. Otherwise, you might chill your back and develop muscle spasms. These neoprene "belly bands" are also used to help lose weight. Remember, you will only lose water weight—not fat weight. In any event, don't continue to rely on a back brace—develop strong muscles.

A new brace that has been successfully used with athletes is the Boston brace. This is made of polyethylene foam and is custom made for each person. As with other braces, it works to flatten the curve of the lower back. This brace is desirable because it allows you to exercise relatively normally.

Coping with Back Pain

If you have trouble with your back, develop a systematic program for rehabilitation. Do your exercises a minimum of five days a week. Write down the exercises you do in a training diary or notebook and keep track of your progress. Start off slowly and gradually increase the intensity of your exercise sessions. Ice massage before and after exercise will make your rehabilitation program more effective.

Observe good habits of posture and body mechanics. When sitting in a chair, make sure your back is erect. Keep your seat forward when you drive your car so that your body is erect. On long auto trips, stop and walk around every one to two hours. When sleeping or standing, avoid postures that cause your lower back to arch. Sleep on a firm mattress—putting a board under the mattress can help provide firm support. Regular exercise is critical to prevent the recurrence of back pain once it disappears. Swimming is a particularly good exercise if you are prone to back pain. Never become complacent—you have to do the exercises outlined in this chapter for the rest of your life; the alternative is a painful back.

Tail Bone Injury

Bruises to the tail bone or coccyx can be very painful and can take a long time to heal. These injuries can occur in any situation where you fall down on your coccyx. In sports such as sledding or tobogganing, where you're already sitting down, these injuries are common; a sudden bounce on the sled can lead to a very painful tail bone. If you sustain a particularly jolting injury of this nature, or if the pain is persistent, see a physician for an x-ray examination. Initially, the injury should be treated with ice massage accompanied by rest for a day or so. Heat and ice contrast treatments can begin after a few days. Heat in the form of a whirlpool bath is relaxing and will help dissipate some of the pain.

Hip Pain

The hip is a well protected joint surrounded by and encased within large and powerful muscles. Because of its large surface area, it is subject to bumps and bruises. Overuse injuries, although less common than in other joints, can occur in the hip joint. Bursitis is common in the hips of runners and joggers.

Bruises

A variety of sports can subject the boney part of your hip to trauma. This injury is prevalent in contact sports, but it can also occur in sports like skiing or skateboarding if you fall on ice or cement. For that matter, you can injure a hip by colliding with a wall or your opponent in sports like racquetball. This injury can drastically affect your sports performance because the hips are vital for movement. It's difficult even to walk without aggravating a hip injury.

The hip should be x-rayed for a possible broken bone. Ice massage or an ice pack is helpful both as an immediate treatment and throughout rehabilitation. Because of the muscle spasms that usually accompany this injury, it's important that you try to maintain some of the range of motion in the joint (muscle spasms will decrease joint flexibility). Do this without putting your weight on your leg (see the range of motion exercises, page 116). Get some rest. After a few days of ice massage, you can begin heat treatment (hot bath or whirlpool). However, because of the large amount of soft tissue in the area, don't begin the heat treatment until most of the pain and swelling have dissipated. Using heat too soon may aggravate the injury. Try to avoid returning to any kind of contact sport or activity that could irritate your hip until the injury is healed.

Muscle Strains

Like other muscle groups, your hip muscles can be overwhelmed and injured in sports and exercise. The treatment for hip muscle injuries is similar to that of other muscle strains.

● Ice and rest. Ice massage is probably the most effective treatment because of the large surface area of the hip. Because of the importance of the hip muscles in movement, rest is important. Try to use a cane or crutches to remove some of the pressure caused by your body weight.

● Try to maintain range of motion in the joint. Initially you can do this in a swimming pool by submerging yourself and moving your leg in large, circular motions. Do these movements in both clockwise and counterclockwise directions.

•As your hip starts to feel better, you can begin hip flexibility exercise outside of the water.

LATERAL HIP STRETCHER This is the best flexibility exercise for this area. Stand about one to two feet from a wall. Lean your upper arm against the wall and press your pelvis inward. You should feel a stretch in your hip muscles. This exercise sometimes helps with back pain as well.

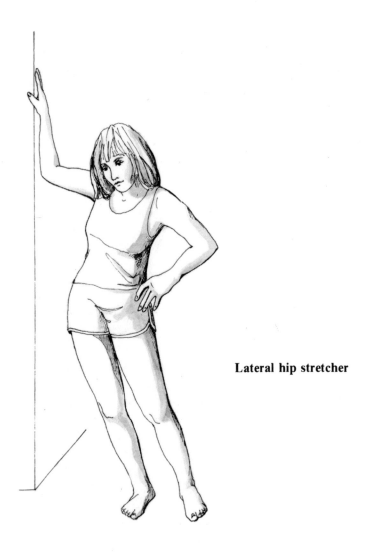

Lateral hip stretcher

SWIVEL HIPS This is another good range of motion exercise. Stand with your feet about shoulder width apart and move your legs and hips in a circular motion—first clockwise, then counterclockwise.

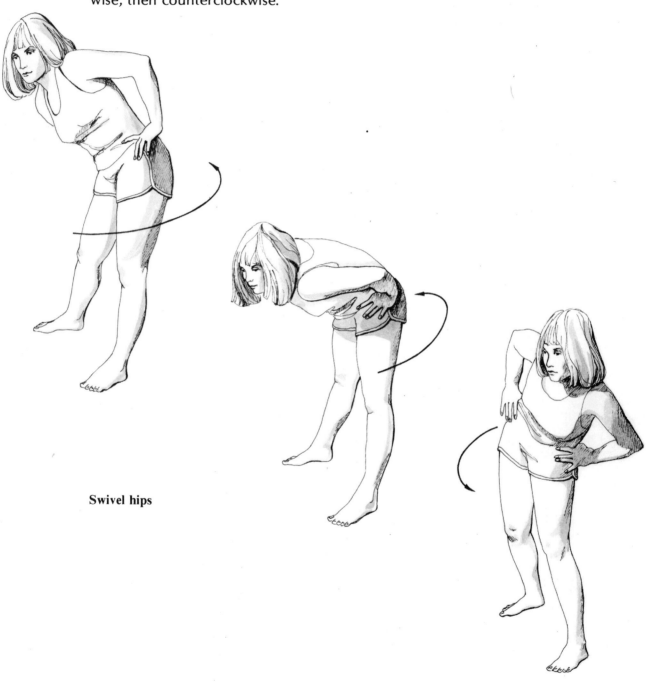

Swivel hips

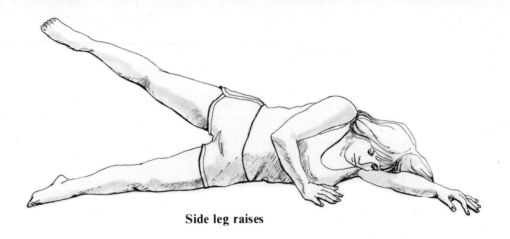

Side leg raises

SIDE LEG RAISES These will help you maintain joint mobility and strength. Lie on your side, with one leg on top of the other. Raise the upper leg, then return it to the starting position. This movement is called hip abduction. You can increase the difficulty of this exercise by wearing a weighted boot or sandbags made from socks. In sports medicine rehabilitation facilities there are machines such as the Cybex that help you to increase the strength of your hip abductors.

HIP ABDUCTION FROM A BAR Hang from a bar and raise both legs sideways simultaneously.

Hip abduction from a bar

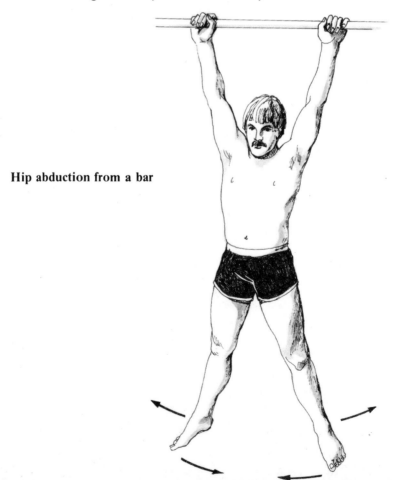

•Don't try to return to sports such as running, skiing, or tennis too early. Start with minimal weight bearing sports such as cycling or swimming. When you're ready to return to sports, begin by running in the shallow end of a pool so that you can break in those hip muscles gradually.

Overuse Injuries

Long distance running and other sports can result in hip pain. Hip pain can sometimes be referred from the back. This means that the problem is really in the back, but you feel it in the hips. Paying close attention to posture, general fitness, and strength and flexibility in the back, hips, stomach, and legs is important in avoiding this problem.

Sometimes the only way to treat hip pain related to heavy training is with trial and error methods and a little patience. First, try changing the brand of shoe you're wearing. Running on hard surfaces may sometimes cause the problem. Try running on a grassy area such as a golf course. Differences in leg length may contribute to hip pain. Try a heel lift, or consult a foot doctor for more precise treatment. Cut down on the intensity of your training—sometimes you can overwhelm your body. Improvements in fitness and condition require only small increments of increased intensity. When you overtrain, your body is telling you to lay off. Listen to your body.

Overuse injuries in the hips are sometimes accompanied by a cracking, grinding sensation in the joint. This is caused by inflammation in the joint. Stretching (see the hip exercises, page 114), rest, and ice will help this condition a lot. Your doctor may be able to prescribe medication to help you.

As with other overtraining-related injuries, try another sport for a while. This way, you can maintain fitness without further aggravating your injury.

Getting the Wind Knocked Out of You

It's not unusual to see a football player get hit so hard that he gets the wind knocked out of him. This phenomenon is common in recreational sports as well. Collisions with other players or objects can give you that terrifying feeling of having extreme breathing difficulty. This phenomenon is caused by a blow to your solar plexus, a collection of nerves in your upper abdomen. The blow causes your large breathing muscle, the diaphragm, to go into spasm. If this happens to you, try to relax. Take short breaths in and long breaths out of your mouth. In most cases this condition passes within a few minutes. If you're with someone who isn't recovering, mouth-to-mouth resuscitation may be necessary.

Rib Injuries

Rib injuries, because of possible lung involvement, should always be evaluated by a physician. Bruised ribs should be handled like other injuries of this nature. Ice and rest are your best bet for the optimal rate of rehabilitation. If your ribs need support to help you return to sports, you can purchase commercially available rib belts.

A good exercise to prevent adhesions in the area is to stretch both of your hands over your head as high as possible. You can also do this exercise by first stretching one arm, then the other. When you injure your ribs, try to avoid contact and collision sports. With conservative treatment, your ribs will heal quickly.

Jogger's Nipples and Cooper's Droopers

Jogger's nipples is an injury that has received notice in an issue of *Time* magazine as something that bugs many runners, both male and female. The condition is caused by friction from a shirt or bra. To prevent this problem, I suggest protecting your nipples with a band-aid or piece of tape, or coating them with petroleum jelly.

Years of running braless or with inadequate support may lead to sagging breast tissue. This condition has been aptly named Cooper's droopers, after Dr. Kenneth Cooper—author of *Aerobics* and the father of our present running craze. Joan Gillette, a trainer for the Virginia Slims Women's Professional Tennis tour, has studied this phenomenon in great detail. Using high speed film, she found that unsupported breasts create a force between 70–110 pounds against the chest during running. She feels it's absolutely essential that women, particularly large breasted women, get adequate support if they are going to run. She found that bras typically found in department stores are inadequate for the demands of sport. She recommends purchasing a custom-made sports bra, manufactured by companies such as Gym Bra (Van Nuys, CA). These bras provide support while allowing freedom of movement.

Side Pains While Running

A pain in the side encountered while running is sometimes called a stitch. Almost every person, at one time or another, has experienced it. The cause is unknown. Some possible causes include intestinal gas and spasm in your breathing muscles. Side pains are prevalent in untrained people, but I've seen even seasoned runners get them in a big race.

There are many things you can try when these pains occur. First, you can try to bite the bullet. Sometimes the pain will go away by itself. Resting for a few minutes helps some people; often the pain will be gone when you start up again. Some experts suggest forcefully expiring through pursed lips while bending at the waist. Belly breathing, taking deep breaths while running, may be a possible remedy. Having an adequate bowel movement before exercising may help if your pains are gas related.

Pains in the center of your chest or in your neck, shoulders, and arms may be symptomatic of angina pectoris. Angina is caused by a relative lack of blood flow through the coronary arteries, which supply your heart with blood. Don't take any chances; severe chest pains may be a sign of trouble. See your doctor immediately if you're having this problem.

Neck Pain

Injuries to the neck sustained in sports can be potentially tragic and should be dealt with with extreme caution. I have seen several young people sustain spinal cord injuries in their upper vertebrae and then become quadriplegics. If you observe a person with a neck injury, don't attempt to move him. You could make the situation much worse. Always consult a physician about a neck injury because the possible consequences are too serious if you don't. Serious injuries to the neck that occur in competitive contact sports such as football are beyond the scope of this book. This discussion will concentrate on neck pain resulting from muscle strains encountered in recreational sports and exercise.

Your head is supported by the bones of your neck and their muscles and ligaments. Because the neck is a relatively narrow base of support, it is susceptible to injury. Your neck is constructed to provide a considerable amount of movement. However, in sports your neck is sometimes subjected to a range of motion that goes beyond the normal. Sudden snaps, violent twists, or overexertion can overwhelm your neck muscles causing pain and injury. Neck injuries are characterized by muscle spasm and painful movement.

Like lower back pain, neck pain can be related to posture as well as movement-related trauma. Your neck has many pain-sensitive nerves that react to abnormal stresses placed upon it. Preventing neck injuries involves maintaining strong, flexible muscles and minimizing nervous tension.

Posture and Neck Pain

Deviations in posture anywhere along your spine, such as in your lower back, may affect your neck. To maintain a proper erect posture, the curves of your spine must remain balanced. An abnormality in one part of the spine will necessarily affect the other parts. So, it's crucial to maintain good whole-body fitness. You may be unaware of the extent to which the different parts of the body are related to each other. It is conceivable that by exercising to prevent back pain, you may indirectly prevent a neck injury.

Your frame of mind affects the postural position of your neck and head as it does with lower back position. If you lack confidence and constantly assume a dejected attitude, you may let your shoulders droop and your head fall forward. This posture forces your neck muscles to support the weight of your head in an incorrect position. These muscles will be constantly fatigued if you do this, thus subject to injury.

A good head and neck posture involves keeping your head up and back and keeping your chin in. Avoid positions that cause you to round your shoulders or increase the curve of your upper spine (cervical vertebrae).

Poor posture of the neck and head is related to some kinds of headache. If you are under a lot of pressure or tension and you have poor posture, this problem can be very difficult to deal with. It's important that you understand some of the bad habits associated with neck pain and work to correct them.

●Try to develop a positive attitude about yourself. Be proud of what you have and who you are. Appreciate yourself—after all, you're all you've got.

• Take time each day to relax. You owe this to yourself. Sit back in a nice, quiet place, close your eyes, and think pleasant thoughts.

• Get enough exercise. Regular exercise will help you relax and can increase pride in yourself. You will have more energy and be able to sleep much easier.

• Concentrate on posture. Think about keeping your head up and shoulders back. You have to develop new, good habits to replace those old slouchy ones. A good exercise to improve neck posture is to put a book or sandbag on your head. To keep these objects from falling, you have to have good posture. (Do this exercise in the privacy of your home or your friends may call you "old sandbag-head.")

• Develop good strength and flexibility in your neck muscles. Below are some exercises that will help.

Sprains and Strains of the Neck

Strains are injuries to neck muscles, while sprains are ligament injuries. Once again, see a physician for any serious injury of this nature. Neck injuries are potentially dangerous and should be treated with extreme caution.

Treatment of these injuries is similar to that of other soft tissue disabilities:

• Ice massage during the early stages of recovery.

• Accompany the ice massage with range of motion exercises. Have someone help you with the ice massage and the exercises. Gently move your head from one side, then to the other. If your injury is serious, do not begin range of motion exercises until you have checked with your physician.

• After a few days, you can also begin heat treatments. Alternate between ice and heat treatments. Heat treatments can include a hot bath, whirlpool, or wet heat pack.

• As your neck improves begin a vigorous program to restore normal range of motion. Apply ice massage before and after your workout—this will increase the effectiveness of your exercises. Start by turning your head to the left and then to the right. Then, nod your head up and then down. Roll both your head and neck around in a circle. First clockwise, then counterclockwise. Do all of these exercises slowly and gradually. Although some pain is inevitable, don't push so hard that you aggravate your injury. However, you must do your exercises in spite of some pain or the injury will take much longer to heal.

●Your doctor may prescribe a neck brace. This will help you support your injured and ailing muscles and ligaments. However, don't rely on this brace indefinitely. Develop strong, flexible muscles—then you won't need a brace.

●Don't return to sports too soon. Try to rehabilitate your neck and avoid a relapse. Rehabilitate your neck slowly with rest, ice, and range of motion exercises.

●Begin neck strengthening exercises as soon as the pain has disappeared. Initially, have someone provide resistance to your neck movements. Have this person place one hand on each side of your head. Move your head to the left and then to the right. Then, have this person provide resistance to your moving your head up and down and laterally from one side to the other. Begin these exercises with a minimum of resistance—then increase the pressure very gradually.

You can purchase a head harness at a sports store that will help strengthen your neck muscles. Place this harness on your head and attach weights to the end of the chain. The harness will provide resistance to neck movements.

A neck harness provides resistance to neck movements.

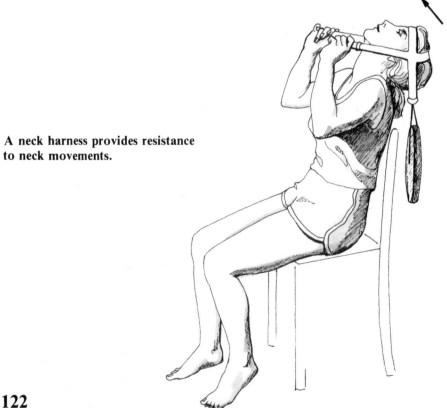

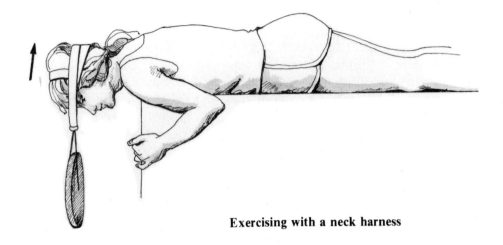

Exercising with a neck harness

Probably the best neck rehabilitation system available is manufactured by Nautilus. They make three different machines that help develop a variety of different movement patterns. These machines are available at many gymnasiums and sports medicine rehabilitation facilities throughout the country. They provide a rapid and specific method for developing strength in neck muscles.

Avoid doing wrestlers neck bridges—supporting your body weight with your head and feet—if you have a neck injury. These exercises can overload weakened muscles and make your disability worse. Neck bridges are very good exercises for developing strong muscles if you have a healthy neck.

Head Injuries

This discussion of head injuries is limited to relatively minor disabilities occurring in recreational sports: nosebleeds and black eyes. Injuries causing unconsciousness, joint dislocations, or fracture should always be examined by a physician. Serious head injuries are rare in noncontact casual sports. However, we have all experienced a nosebleed or black eye from such activities. It's easy to get hit in the eye with a tennis ball, hit yourself in the head with your own racquet in racquetball, or crash into an opponent in a friendly game of basketball.

Nosebleed

You can get a nosebleed from getting hit in the nose by another person or object. Some people experience this condition by blowing the nose too vigorously or from exposure to the cold, dry air of the mountains. This is a relatively minor problem that disappears quickly if handled properly. After fifteen to thirty minutes you can usually return to play. The problem looks a lot worse than it is. The biggest annoyance is looking like you came out second in a match with Muhammad Ali. Wash your face and play on.

The treatment for a nosebleed is simple: Lie down in a comfortable position with your head elevated. Squeeze your nose with your thumb and index finger for three to six minutes. Squeeze firmly so that you apply enough pressure to stop the bleeding. Don't stuff gauze or cotton in your nose or under your upper lip as this will delay the clotting mechanisms. After the bleeding has stopped, try not to blow your nose or sneeze for several hours.

If you have difficulty stopping the bleeding, it's best to seek medical help. However, if you apply the necessary pressure to your nose, this shouldn't be necessary. If you suspect a broken nose, it's best to get it x-rayed.

Black Eye

The tissue around your eyes has a very prolific blood supply. A blow to this area can cause internal bleeding and can result in discoloration commonly known as a black eye. The classic treatment for a black eye has always been to place a steak over the injury. With the price of beef rising, this is no longer a viable treatment. The best thing to do is to place an ice pack or wet towel saturated with ice chips over the area for about fifteen minutes. Repeat the cold treatment periodically for twenty-four to forty-eight hours. Avoid blowing your nose or sneezing vigorously after receiving this injury as the internal bleeding may increase, making your black eye blacker.

This injury is somewhat common in racquetball and squash. In an enclosed area, it's easy to get hit in the head in the heat of battle. It's a good idea to wear eye protectors to prevent serious injuries of this nature.

Don't immediately dismiss a black eye as a trivial injury. A blow to the head can sometimes result in fractures of your cheekbone or eye sockets that initially appear quite innocent. Look for any disturbances in your vision such as blurring or an increased sensitivity to light. Pay attention to any changes in the appearance of your eyes. Compare one eye with the other. Are the pupils the same size? Are the irises symmetrical? If a more serious injury is suspected, see an eye doctor immediately.

Instant Replay

- If your spine is properly aligned, little muscle action is required to maintain an erect posture. If you have bad posture, you force your muscles to support your body and thereby increase the risk of a trunk injury.
- To prevent back pain, develop strong abdominal, back, and leg muscles, and flexible back, hip, and hamstring muscles.
- Avoid postures that cause your lower back to arch. Observe proper postures for sitting, standing, and sleeping.
- Regular exercise is essential for a healthy back and trunk.
- Proper posture for your neck and head involves keeping your head aligned over your spine. Prevention of neck pain involves adequate neck and shoulder strength and flexibility, good posture, and minimizing emotional tension and anxiety.
- Muscular–skeletal injuries should be treated with rest, ice massage, and range of motion exercises. Serious trunk and head injuries should be evaluated by a physician.

6.

INJURIES TO THE SHOULDERS, ARMS, AND HANDS

When I was a young discus thrower, my coach summarized the principles of discus technique with the phrase: "hip, whip, flip." Although that sounds pretty bizarre if you're not familiar with track and field, it has an application to many recreational sports requiring upper body movements. My coach was trying to tell me to use my whole body to propel the discus. In sports such as tennis or softball, you can't let your arm and shoulder do all the work either or you'll get an injury. You have to concentrate on the proper transition of force or injuries are almost inevitable.

The majority of upper body injuries in recreational sports are related to overuse—although traumatic injuries are not uncommon. Overuse injuries of the upper extremities are related to several factors: poor technique, inappropriate equipment, lack of adequate strength and flexibility, and poor training habits. Failure to prevent upper body injuries results in what is known in the locker room as "a bad wing." Proper training and exercise habits are essential if you are to avoid pain in your upper extremities. Make sure you warm up adequately before exerting full effort. In tennis, for example, this means you don't start blasting fireball serves over the net as soon as you get out on the court. Begin on the sidelines with some general stretching exercises; then hit a few ground strokes for a while. As your arm gets warmed up, you can start serving. Go through a few nice and easy, then gradually increase the intensity. When you are warmed up, you can deliver a series of sizzlers to your dazzled opponent without sustaining an arm injury. The same thing is true of throwing a softball or football. Start off easy for a few throws— then gradually increase the intensity and distance.

There has been somewhat of a de-emphasis recently on strength development among casual sportspersons with the rise in popularity of running. Running develops cardiovascular endurance which has been shown to be the most important factor of physical fitness. Cardiovascular fitness is indeed important when you consider the role of endurance capacity in reducing heart disease, but a lack of upper body strength may increase your risk of injury in arm and shoulder sports such as tennis. Cardiovascular fitness doesn't replace strength; you need both. If you are going to play upper body sports, you should work to systematically increase the strength in your shoulders and arms. You can increase strength with various calisthenic exercises and resistive exercises with weights (see page 139) or with exercise machines such as the Universal Gym, Nautilus, or Cybex. Your increased strength will not only result in less chance of injury, but it will help you develop a rifle serve that will inspire both awe and fear in your opponent. Remember, if they can't see it, they can't hit it.

Shoulder Injuries

Your shoulder joint is important in just about every sport. If you aren't using it directly for throwing a ball or a frisbee, you're using it for balance in sports such as ice skating. The joint is particularly susceptible to injury because of its anatomy. Unlike the hip joint's, the shoulder's boney attachments are shallow. However, the shoulder's anatomy allows an incredible range of movement. Because the shoulder joint is dominated by soft tissue, it is a likely site for sports injuries. The tendons of the joint can become irritated by overuse in sports such as tennis, swimming, and softball; sudden traumatic injuries, such as falling on an outstretched arm, can irritate your shoulder bursa—the fluid-filled sacs that reduce joint friction—causing a lot of pain. Pain in the shoulder has a tendency to make you decrease movement; this in turn makes joint mobility more difficult. As a rule, if you don't fully use a joint, you will lose a certain amount of its range of motion. Perhaps more than with any other joint, your handling of a shoulder injury will ultimately determine whether you improve rapidly or develop chronic pain.

Shoulder movements are accomplished with the help of a number of joints—the glenohumeral, sternoclavicular, the acromioclavicular, and the coracoclavicular. Strictly speaking, this area should be referred to as the shoulder girdle. Normal function includes smooth, effortless, and synchronous movements of all parts of this shoulder girdle. Improper sports techniques, weak and inflexible muscles, or nervous tension may cause an injury.

Several serious injuries to the shoulder girdle are possible—dislocations and separations, bone breaks, and tears in tissue. A natural reaction of many people is to try to break a fall with an outstretched arm. This can be an unfortunate reflex—you may get a broken arm or dislocated or separated shoulder as a result of it. Obviously, a broken arm should be treated by a physician. So should a separated or dislocated shoulder. You should not attempt to reset a dislocated or separated shoulder. When these injuries occur, there is typically extensive muscle spasm in the area. By trying to reset the shoulder, you may break a bone or damage the nerves or blood supply to the area. Other serious injuries to the shoulder include tears in the connective tissue structure of the joint. You should seek medical help (preferably an orthopedic specialist) for any serious shoulder injury.

Since most shoulder injuries in sports are related to overuse, faulty techniques, and poor training habits, and are not the serious, traumatic injuries described above, a physician may be of little help other than to provide sympathy and rehabilitation exercises. As a general rule, if your shoulder doesn't improve in one to two weeks or if you're feeling excessive pain, see your physician. Otherwise, follow the appropriate procedure for shoulder rehabilitation beginning on page 130.

The most common sports-related shoulder injuries are tendonitis, bursitis, and strains. These injuries must be dealt with aggressively to prevent a condition called frozen shoulder, a phenomenon that can easily arise if you let the pain defeat you. This condition is accompanied by local swelling—movements become painful and restricted. Frozen shoulder occurs most frequently in people over thirty years of age. The progression follows a common path:

• Your shoulder is injured. You experience muscle spasm and pain. You are afraid to move your arm because it hurts. You keep your movements to a minimum.

• Disuse of your shoulder only serves to make things worse. Movements that only a few months before were commonplace have become excruciatingly painful. Adhesions have formed in your shoulder girdle that make motion difficult. Lack of motion has led to restriction of your movements.

You must keep your ailing shoulder mobile and maintain its range of motion or your injury will get worse; you might risk having chronic, permanent pain.

If you're tense and have a low pain threshold, you are more susceptible to frozen shoulder. Get psyched! Maintain motion. When you strain a shoulder muscle or develop bursitis, keep that shoulder moving, even if it hurts a little. Ice will act as a partial anesthetic. It will allow you to exercise in spite of small hurts but will not mask the pain that tells you when you are pushing too far.

Like other injuries of the upper body, shoulder injuries can be related to faulty posture and body mechanics. If your shoulders are hunched over, the possible joint motions are restricted and tendons can become irritated. With time the connective tissue begins to deteriorate, causing pain. You must work hard to maintain efficient body position, and work regularly to develop strong and flexible shoulder muscles.

Shoulder Tendonitis

Repeated abuse of the shoulder joint can inflame shoulder tendons. This injury is prevalent in sports such as swimming, tennis, and baseball that require shoulder movements with the arms raised to the level of the head or above. The injury may be accompanied by swelling and local tissue damage due to the repeated trauma. If the condition is allowed to continue, the initial inflammation will be accompanied by calcium deposits on the tendon and bursitis (see page 132). Lack of movement because of pain may result in shoulder adhesions that will further restrict your movements.

Treatment should be aimed at regaining full range of motion and good muscle strength. Return to full sports participation with caution. Ideally, you should wait until your shoulder is pain free. Proper care of shoulder tendonitis is essential to avoid permanent shoulder pain.

• Initial treatment should include rest from the activity causing the irritation for at least two days. Rest, however, doesn't mean immobilizing your shoulder. You must begin range of motion exercises immediately. When I say to rest, I mean to avoid excessively traumatic movements such as tennis serves and overhead throwing motions. An arm sling will help remove some of the stresses of gravity from your shoulder.

• Apply ice massage periodically for at least two days. Rub the ice over a large area for about ten minutes. Initially, an ice pack anchored with an elastic bandage is adequate.

• Begin mobility exercises immediately (see page 134). In performing range of motion exercises for an injured shoulder you have to walk a fine line: you must move your shoulder in spite of some pain and stiffness but not to the point where the pain becomes excessive. If you push too hard, you will cause muscle spasms and your shoulder flexibility will actually decrease. Move your shoulder to the point that you feel sharp pain, then don't go any further. Remember, there is a distinction between stiffness and minor irritation, and sharp pain. Minor pain is to be expected and overcome, continued movements with sharp pain can make your shoulder worse. Using ice massage before and after your range of motion exercises can greatly facilitate the process and minimize muscle spasms.

• If you have a tendency to develop shoulder tendonitis, modify your sports techniques and training procedures. Always warm up before you play. It makes little sense to go out on the field and try to throw a ball as far as you can. Begin with some shoulder stretching and mobility exercises. Then, gradually increase the intensity of your movements. Avoid movements that cause pain. When you throw a baseball or softball, try to throw with more of a sidearm movement than one coming directly overhead. Many swimmers develop a painful shoulder because they breathe only on one side—try breathing on both sides. In racquetball, try to keep the number of ceiling shots to a minimum. In tennis, make sure your side is facing the net when you serve. Try to use more of a slice serve—this will place less strain on your shoulders. In most sports, try to use your whole body rather than making your arm do all the work.

In general, try to restrict your movements to below shoulder level as much as possible. In tennis and racquetball, this means trying to make contact with the ball closer to the ground. In skiing, this means not flailing your poles about as you come down the slope.

●Don't let your arm get cold after you play. Put on a warm-up jacket or sweat shirt. After exercise your muscles are more susceptible to spasm from the cooling effect of your sweat. Although this may seem contradictory, an ice massage on a sore shoulder after a game may be helpful. The ice massage will prevent muscle spasm. Postexercise stretching will also prevent spasms and joint stiffness.

●As pain disappears, work to strengthen your shoulder muscles. Strong muscles are less easily injured. You can strengthen your shoulder muscles with weight exercises or upper body calisthenics. (See page 139.)

●Heat treatments, in addition to ice massage, can begin two to three days after the initial symptoms. A hot whirlpool bath will not only relax your shoulder, but will provide a good environment for range of motion exercises. A good whirlpool exercise is to bend at the waist with your arm and shoulder submerged in the water. Gently make large arm circles—first clockwise, then counterclockwise. Other forms of heat treatment such as hydrocollator packs and hot towels are good for this type of injury, too. If your shoulder is swollen or painful to the touch, it's best to avoid heat treatments for a few days. Ice is always better during the initial stages of soft tissue injury.

●Massage is sometimes soothing for tendonitis in the shoulder. Try to direct your massage motion toward the heart. Avoid massage during the first few days because of the danger of interfering with the rehabilitation process.

●Aspirin may help relieve some of the inflammation.

Bursitis

Bursitis is another common shoulder ailment. Shoulder bursa are fluid-filled sacs that reduce friction in the joint. Shoulder bursitis can occur if you jam your arm into your shoulder joint or fall on an outstretched arm in a sport like skiing or soccer. Repeated trauma to the shoulder in sports such as tennis and softball may also aggravate your shoulder bursa.

Regular application of ice massage or an ice pack for the first forty-eight hours after the initial symptoms will help to minimize pain and any swelling. After the first few days of cold treatment, you can begin heat applications—hot packs, hot baths, or whirlpool baths. Be sure to do range of motion exercises in the bath. Avoid raising your arms over your head as this movement may impinge upon your shoulder bursa and aggravate them. Aspirin may help to reduce the inflammation.

Rest is important for early recovery from shoulder bursitis. Try to participate in sports that place minimal demands upon your shoulders. Decrease participation in sports such as swimming and tennis that force you to extend your arms, until your shoulder feels better. If you ski or ride a skateboard, learn how to fall. Falling on a straight arm, in addition to aggravating shoulder bursa, may result in a broken arm or dislocated shoulder. Try to roll when you fall instead of forcing your shoulder to absorb the entire weight of your body. Learning the techniques of judo or gymnastics may help you learn these skills. Be sure to receive instruction from a qualified teacher.

Sprains and Strains of the Shoulder

Sprains and strains to the shoulders can result from acute injury—when you fall on an outstretched arm, from overwhelming your shoulder muscles in sports such as weight lifting, or from repeated small injuries—when you pitch a baseball or serve a tennis ball. You can prevent these injuries by developing proper sports techniques for falling, serving, and throwing; maintaining good shoulder strength and flexibility; and observing the principles of training.

Particularly among males, there is a machismo associated with strong shoulder muscles. Women also are recognizing the value of strength in their sports programs. Many people try to rush their progress—doing too much too soon. Lifting more weight than you can handle can easily subject you to an injury. You are much better off taking it slow and easy. Warming up is critical for your shoulder muscles because of the joint's capacity for movement. Before playing a sport that requires upper body movements, warm your shoulder up thoroughly. Keep warm with a sweat suit or windbreaker until your shoulders are ready for action.

The treatment for shoulder strains and sprains is similar to treatment for other strains and sprains.

●Use ice, in the form of an ice pack or ice massage, immediately and for the first two to three days after the injury.

●Rest your shoulder but begin range of motion exercises right away. The shoulder is very susceptible to the formation of adhesions that can result in "frozen shoulder" if mobility is not maintained.

●Alternate between heat and cold treatments after two to three days. You will find your exercise sessions are more beneficial if you apply ice massage before and after your workout.

●After much of the pain has disappeared, begin shoulder strengthening exercises (see page 139). Make sure to perform these exercises through a full range of motion. Because of the many movement patterns possible in the shoulder girdle, you have to do a variety of exercises. Strength is specific—that is, developing the muscles responsible for one shoulder movement will not necessarily develop strength in another shoulder muscle.

●Don't return to active sports participation until your shoulder is completely rehabilitated. Remember, your shoulder is supported mainly by soft tissue. Muscles, tendons, and ligaments are easily irritated if they are stressed before they are fully healed.

Shoulder Bruises

The deltoid, the curved muscle on your upper arm, is easily bruised in sports. Collisions with people or objects, or falls can cause this injury. Because of the large amount of soft tissue in the shoulder, bruises can be debilitating to your sports participation. Ice the area immediately. Placing a plastic bag filled with ice on your shoulder and wrapping it with an elastic bandage will work quite well. Continue icing the area periodically until the pain disappears. Make sure to maintain range of motion in your shoulder. After three days, you can perform your mobility exercises in a hot tub or whirlpool. Avoid active sports participation for one to three days, depending upon the amount of pain you're experiencing. Don't use aspirin for about a week after this injury—aspirin affects your blood's ability to clot and may make the injury worse.

Backpacker's Palsy

This condition is characterized by numbness and pain in your shoulder and arm, particularly on your nondominant side (if you are right handed, left is your nondominant side). It is caused by the pressure of pack straps on nerves in your shoulders. Backpacker's palsy can last anywhere from an hour or so to several weeks. The damage is usually never permanent. It may cause muscle weakness and make you wish you had taken the bus instead of walked. Another related problem is swelling in your hands and forearms—also caused by pack straps.

You can avoid this problem by purchasing a good pack. Good backpacks, such as the classic Kelty, place more of the weight on your hips than on your shoulders. Don't carry too much weight. Rest often and stretch your arms over your head. If you're feeling a lot of pain, discontinue backpacking or get someone else to carry your stuff such as a mule or mule-like friend.

Shoulder Exercises

The first shoulder exercises you try following an injury should be aimed at maintaining the range of motion in the joint. Initially, you should avoid exercises that cause you to raise your arms over your head—these movements can cause impingement of soft tissue by bone. You will get more from your exercises by preceding them with ice massage to your shoulder. After the first few days, you can do some of your exercises in a whirlpool bath, hot tub, or swimming pool. Perform the range of motion exercises daily. When most of the pain has disappeared, you can begin shoulder strengthening exercises. Work gradually but consistently in developing shoulder strength. Weakened muscles are easily reinjured if pushed too far. Muscle strength and flexibility are particularly important in the shoulder because of its dependence upon soft tissue for support.

Range of Motion Exercises

Do these exercises two to three times during the day. Perform ten to fifty repetitions during each session.

PENDULUM EXERCISES These are excellent during the early stages of recovery since they allow you to develop and maintain range of motion without irritating your shoulder muscles, tendons, and bursa. Bend over at the

Pendulum exercise

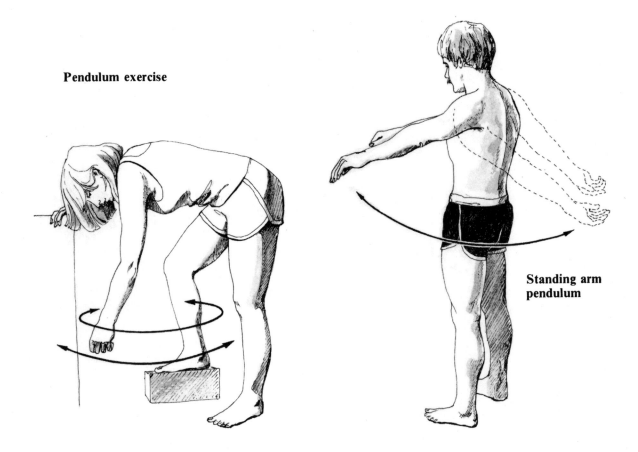

Standing arm pendulum

waist, bending your knees slightly. If you want, you can rest your head on a high stool and prop your foot up on a block. Let your injured arm dangle. Move your arm, with elbow straight, in a circle—first clockwise, then counter-clockwise. Then, move your arm forward, then backward. (Avoid moving your arm to the side during the early stages of recovery.) Next rotate your arm at the shoulder inward, then outward. You can also do these movements holding a weight.

STANDING ARM PENDULUMS From a standing position with your arms at your sides, bring both arms up in front to shoulder level or just below, return to starting position, then swing arms behind you, relax.

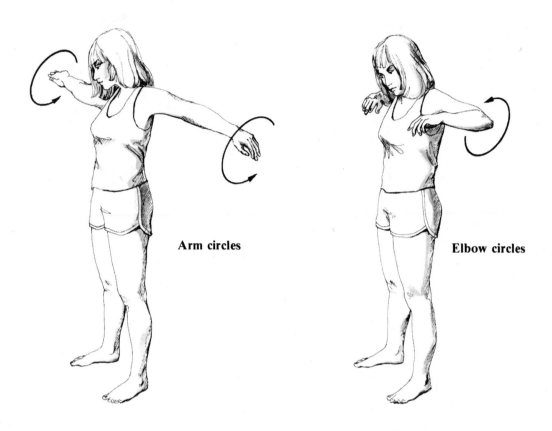

Arm circles   Elbow circles

ARM CIRCLES Stand with your arms extended at your sides. Face your palms downward. Begin the exercises by making small arm circles forward, then backward. Gradually increase the circumference of the arm circles. Also do this exercise with your palms facing upwards.

ELBOW CIRCLES Stand with your elbows bent, upper arms horizontal, or with your hands behind your head, fingers interlocked, elbows extended to the side. Circle your elbows forward, then backward.

SHOULDER SHRUGS Shrug your shoulders upward, then rotate them forward and backward.

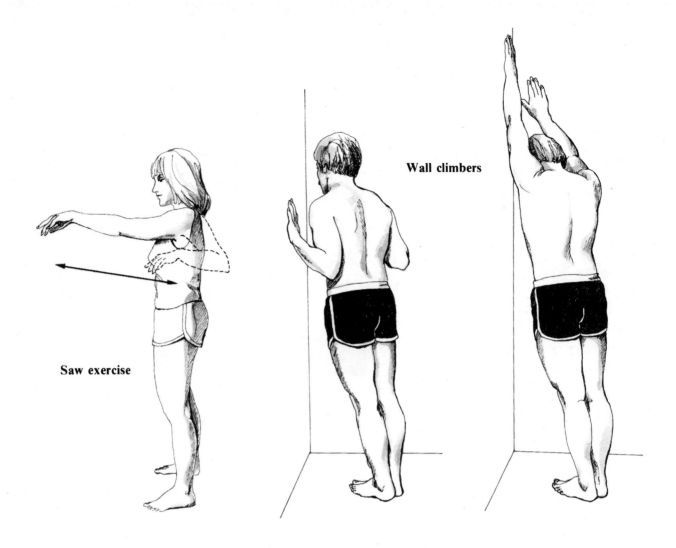

Saw exercise

Wall climbers

SAW EXERCISE From a standing position, bend your elbow and hold an imaginary saw in your hand. Push the saw forward then backward, concentrating on getting as much shoulder movement as possible.

WALL CLIMBERS Lean against a wall at an angle with your arms straight and extended upwards. Bring your head closer to the wall by moving your hands up the wall.

BAR HANGING As your shoulder injury begins to heal, you can begin overhead exercises that place more strain on your soft tissue. Find a relatively high chin-up bar and hang from it. Remain in a hanging position for ten to thirty seconds. This exercise develops both strength and flexibility.

Towel circles

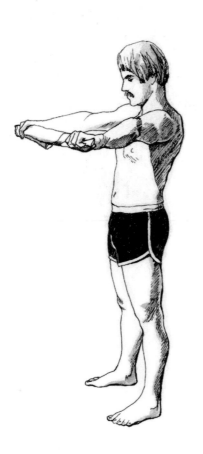 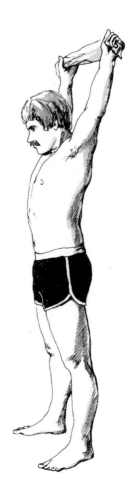

TOWEL CIRCLES This one is for people who are starting to feel pretty good and are anxious to return to the playing field. Grasp a towel at both ends and extend your arms in front of you. Raise your arms as high over your head as you can. Continue to circle your arms behind you until the towel is touching your low back. Then, reverse the exercise, bringing the towel over your head to the front. As your flexibility increases, gradually move your hand placements closer to the middle of the towel. If you have a history of shoulder dislocation, consult your physician before doing this one.

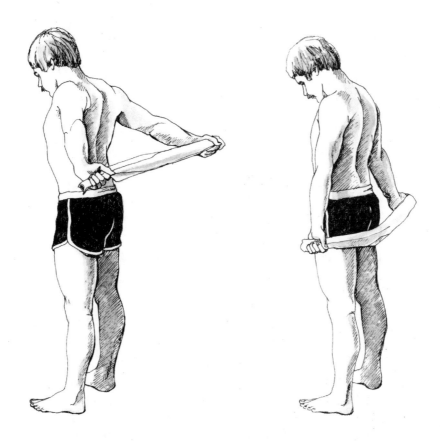

Shoulder Strengthening Exercises

There are three basic types of shoulder strengthening exercises that will develop the shoulder joint.

- Resistance exercises using your own body weight
- Resistance exercises using weights, pulleys, or elastic
- Resistance exercises using exercise machines

The exercise possibilities in the shoulder joint are tremendously varied, reflecting the movement patterns of the shoulder itself. Adequate strengthening of this joint should include as many movements as possible. Vigorous pursuit of strong shoulder muscles will help you prevent, or at least minimize, further shoulder pain.

The next group of exercises uses your own body weight as resistance.

PUSH-UPS Start with a push-up variation. Lean against a wall with your hands, then push yourself from the wall. As your shoulders become stronger, increase the angle of your body. Progress to the standard push-up positions. You can begin with modified floor push-ups—assume a four point position with both your knees and both your hands on the ground. Keeping your back straight, lower your chest to the ground, then push your body back up to the starting position. Next, support your weight on your toes and hands. Keeping legs and back straight, lower your chest to the ground, then push up.

PULL-UPS Hang from a chin-up bar and pull yourself up until your chin goes over the top. Lower yourself slowly. You can do this exercise in a number of ways: with your hands grasping the bar, palms facing you or facing away; with a wide or narrow grip; or behind the neck, bringing the back of your head to the bar. If you have trouble doing this exercise, begin by just hanging from the bar and trying to increase the amount of time you can hang. Next, make repeated efforts to pull yourself up. Even if you don't succeed, you will begin to develop strength by making the effort. Have someone assist you with the exercise by grabbing your legs just below the knees and helping you up. Pretty soon you won't need any assistance—you will be performing pull-ups with the best of them.

DIPS Parallel bars are the best place to do dips. Stand between the bars. Support your weight between the bars until your upper arms are parallel with the ground. Push yourself back to the starting position.

Weight training exercises are perhaps the best way to strengthen the shoulder girdle. During the early phases of your strengthening program, start off with relatively light weights. Begin with ten to fifteen repetitions. Gradually increase the amount of weight and decrease the

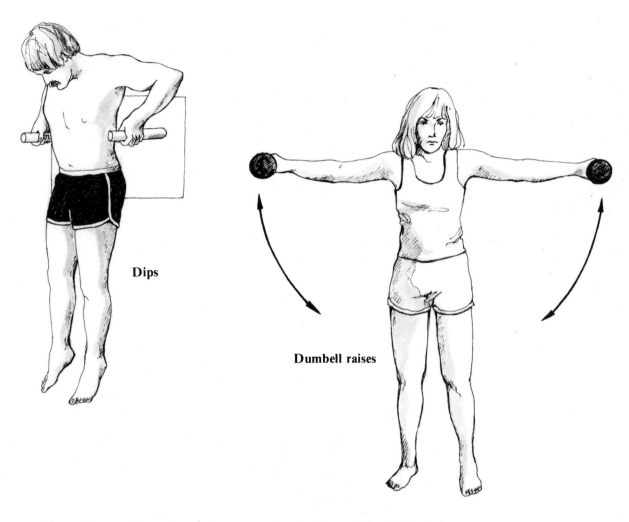

Dips

Dumbell raises

number of repetitions (you decrease the number of repetitions so you can use more weight). After three to six months, you should be performing five to ten repetitions.

DUMBBELL RAISES Grasp the dumbbells and let them hang at your sides with your arms extended. Do this exercise in two planes of movement: to the side, and to the front. First, keeping your arms straight, raise the dumbbells in a sideward plane until both of your hands are over your head. Return to the starting position. Next, raise both dumbbells directly in front of you over your head. You can move both dumbbells simultaneously or one at a time.

Injuries to the Shoulders, Arms, and Hands   **141**

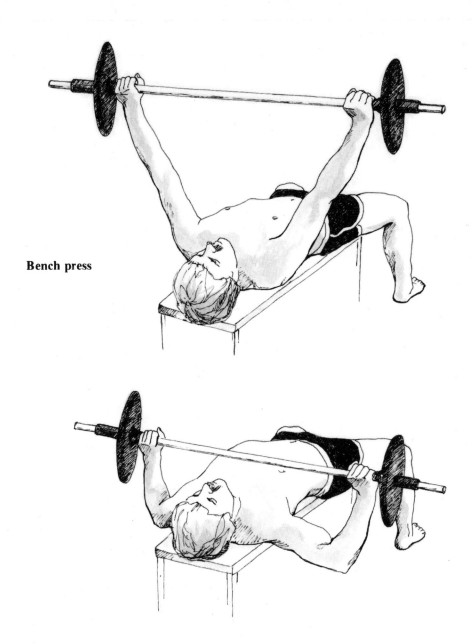

Bench press

BENCH PRESS For this exercise use either a barbell or dumbbells. Lie in a supine position on a bench. Grasp the bar at about shoulder width and support it over your chest. Lower the weight to your chest; then press it back to the starting position. This exercise will develop your shoulders, chest, and arms.

SEATED PRESS Sit on a bench or lean against a slant board. Support the barbell or dumbbell then press the weight over your head; return it to the starting position. It is important to keep your trunk straight so you don't injure your back.

PULLOVERS Lie on your back on a bench with your head either on the bench or hanging over the edge. Grasp a barbell that is placed directly behind your head on the floor. With your elbows bent and close to your head, pull the weight from the floor over your head to your chest. Then, slowly return it to the floor.

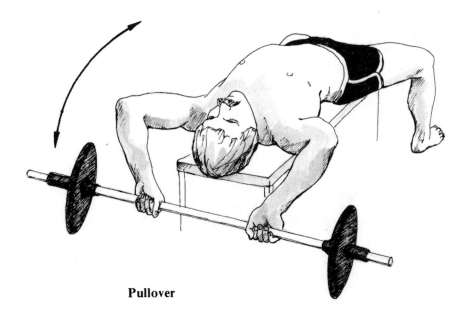

Pullover

SHOULDER SHRUG From a standing position, grasp a barbell and hold it at waist level. Keeping your arms straight, slowly shrug your shoulders—return to the starting position.

Other Shoulder Exercise Possibilities

There are countless other weight training shoulder exercises you can do. I suggest you consult a good strength training book such as *Scientific Principles and Methods of Strength Fitness* by Dr. John O'Shea (Addison-Wesley, 1976).

There are portable strength training devices you can consider. A good, inexpensive device you can buy at a scientific supply house is a length of surgical tubing. Cut a piece about two to three feet long—grasp each end and pull. As you get stronger, place your hands closer to the center of the tube segment. You can buy a three-foot length of tubing for less than one dollar. The possible exercises are limited only by your imagination. Remember, if you add resistance to any movement, you are increasing the strength you can derive from that movement.

There are also various pulley devices that will help you increase your shoulder strength. They are produced by such companies as Exer-Genie and Apollo. They are popular with some professional athletic teams and may be appropriate for the more casual sportsperson. These devices are portable and relatively inexpensive and provide good exercise for your shoulder muscles.

Various manufacturers produce exercise machines specifically designed to develop shoulder strength. Exercises on devices like the Universal Gym and Marcy Gym closely resemble the more traditional weight training exercises such as the shoulder press, bench press, and lat pull. Elaborate devices from other manufacturers, such as Nautilus, develop a large variety of the possible shoulder movements.

If you receive a shoulder injury, you must work hard for complete rehabilitation. You can increase strength and flexibility regardless of the training method you use. Just follow two simple principles: consistently exercise your shoulder through the complete range of motion, and systematically but gradually increase the training load. With hard work you can not only rid yourself of shoulder pain but prevent it in the future.

Returning to Sports Following a Shoulder Injury

There are several techniques you can use to help you return to active sports without reinjuring yourself. These techniques require you to understand the basics of shoulder movement during overhead throwing and racquet motions. The movement phases of throwing a ball and serving a tennis ball are very similar: (1) cock your arm, (2) accelerate the ball or racquet, (3) release or make contact with the ball, (4) follow through. It's during the acceleration and release phases of the motions that injuries occur. If you are not careful to fully rehabilitate your shoulder in strength and flexibility, you will very likely reinjure yourself. The following techniques increase the effectiveness of the acceleration phases of throwing a ball and serving.

Throwing a ball:

● Begin by throwing the ball with a high arc but with relatively little force. This movement forces you to release the ball early and minimizes the pain you'd otherwise feel if you tried to throw the ball with speed or accuracy. Perform this first phase during the first three to five sessions. Rest at least one day between sessions.

● During the second phase, try to throw the ball a little further, with the same trajectory (arc). Be sure to warm your arm up before throwing any great distances. Remember, don't throw the ball in a straight line. This exercise should be practiced a minimum of three to five sessions, with a day's rest between sessions, before you move on.

● During the third phase, lower the trajectory of the ball, but don't yet try for accuracy or great speed. Your throw should look more like a line drive. Practice this exercise for at least three to five sessions.

● During the final phase, you can begin to throw for speed and accuracy. You can release the ball at the proper position and your shoulder should be able to withstand the stresses without reinjury. This last phase is like throwing the ball overhand hard and accurately from the pitcher's mound to home plate.

Tennis serve and overhead: When you return to tennis or racquetball, avoid overhead shots. Perform these drills first to get your shoulder back in shape. I will use the tennis serve as an example, but the same principles hold for racquetball.

● Toss the ball up in the normal fashion. Attempt to serve the ball with a slice, using a slightly sidearm motion. By not serving with an overhead motion, you're placing less stress on your shoulder. Do this exercise for three to five days, ten to twenty serves per day. Rest at least one day between sessions.

• Toss the ball up normally, but this time hit the ball with more of an overhead motion. Don't worry about getting the ball in the service area. Go through a normal service motion without exerting a lot of force. Perform this phase for three days with a day's rest between practice sessions.

• Hit your serves closer to the service area. Go through your normal serving motion with only slightly more force than in phase two.

• Hit the ball with more intensity. Concentrate on good technique and service accuracy.

The progression for racquetball is to stay away from overhead shots initially, then gradually to incorporate them into your game.

Tennis Elbow

Tennis elbow is an overuse injury characterized by pain in the elbow region. Tennis elbow may be inevitable. Take a relatively weak joint such as the elbow and increase the stress on it by exerting a lot of force on an extension of your arm (your tennis racquet) and something's got to give. At least 50 percent of all tennis players experience this injury at one time or another. The methods of treatment have been tremendously varied, ranging from rest and immobilization to surgery.

Tennis elbow is usually caused by injury to the muscles and tendons in the forearm around the outside or lateral part of your elbow (wrist extensors). Although the injury is associated with tennis, it can occur in any activity or occupation that requires a lot of work from forearm muscles. Tennis elbow is prevalent in players over thirty years of age and seems to have to do with a lack of upper body strength, flexibility, and endurance. Equipment is very important; because of its weight, playing with a wooden racquet makes you more susceptible than playing with a steel, aluminum, or fiberglass racquet. String tension and grip size are also involved. Generally speaking, the incidence of this injury is proportional to the frequency and severity of stresses experienced by your forearm muscles.

Research studies have shown tennis elbow to be a complex phenomenon. The longer you play tennis, the more chance you have of developing the problem. Tennis elbow is very common in skilled recreational-level tennis players who play three or more days a week. If you play six to seven days a week, you have more than a 50 percent chance of getting this injury, as opposed to only a 26 percent chance if you play once a week. Expert players are by no means immune—although they are less likely to get tennis elbow than intermediate recreational players, they are more likely to experience the injury than beginning players.

Preventing Tennis Elbow

Tennis elbow can become a chronic condition if you aren't careful. There are many things you can do to prevent this injury:

●Develop good strength, flexibility, and endurance in your arms and shoulders (see shoulder exercises, page 134, and arm exercises, pages 148, 149, and 151). By systematically working on upper body fitness, you can reduce the chances of getting tennis elbow.

●Develop good tennis techniques. The backhand stroke initiates the beginning of elbow pain in many people. An incorrect stroke typically requires that most of the power come from the relatively weak forearm muscles. Try to use your shoulder and body weight in a smooth transition of force. Keep your elbow straight and your weight on your front foot when you hit the ball. You might consider going to a two-handed backhand as this stroke places less strain on your elbow. A person with a good two-handed backhand almost never gets tennis elbow. Try to hit all of your strokes fluidly and smoothly.

●Good and appropriate equipment is important. Use a lighter, more flexible racquet made of aluminum, steel, or fiberglass. Use a large grip—a small grip results in a lot of torque in your forearm and may cause injury. Don't have your racquet strung too tightly—most people should string their racquets between fifty-five and sixty pounds. Unless you play like "Joe Pro," you don't need to string your racquet at sixty-five pounds. A looser string tension will give you better control of your racquet and decrease the trauma to your elbow. Some experts suggest using gut strings because they give more than nylon and thus stress your elbow less.

●Warm up before you attempt a full-effort game. Start off with some stretching exercise, then hit some easy ground strokes, and finally increase the tempo.

●Use new balls. Dead (or wet) balls have less resilience so they increase the tension on your elbow. Maybe you can get your partner to spring for a new can.

●Keep warm—wear a warm-up jacket until you are ready to play. Chilled muscles are easily injured.

Caring for Your Tennis Elbow

The symptoms of tennis elbow may last many months. Your rehabilitation program must include a combination of patience and hard work. Remember, tennis elbow is an overuse injury—therefore, the treatment must include a measure of tender loving care and rest.

●As with other soft tissue injuries, the initial treatment should include ice, compression, and elevation. Put crushed ice or small ice cubes into a plastic bag, place it over the area producing the pain, and wrap it with an elastic bandage. Keep the ice on for about twenty minutes at a time. Repeat this procedure periodically throughout the day. Icing your elbow will minimize both the pain and inflammation associated with the injury.

●During the early stages, you can combine ice with range of motion exercises. Apply ice massage for eight to ten minutes first.

FOREARM SUPINATION AND PRONATION Gently rotate your forearm. First rotate your lower arm so that your palm is facing up (supination); then rotate your forearm so your palm is facing down (pronation). Perform these exercises with your elbow locked and bent. After some of the pain has dissipated, you can add resistance to these movements to help you strengthen your forearm muscles. Put a dumbbell in your hands as you rotate your forearm. These exercises can also be performed isometrically (muscle contraction without movement). Grab an immovable pipe or bar with your palms facing up—isometrically attempt to turn your palms down. Do the same exercise with your palms down—attempt to turn them up.

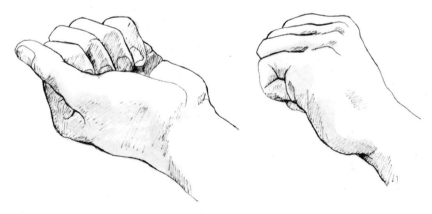

Supination (palm up)   **Pronation (palm down)**

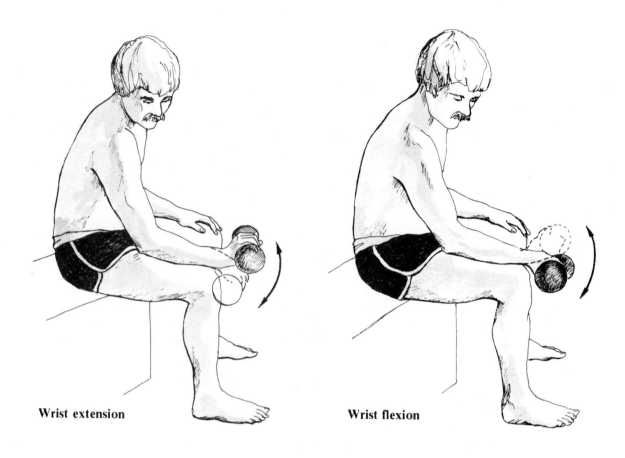

Wrist extension

Wrist flexion

WRIST EXTENSION Put your forearm on a table or on your knee and hang your hand over the edge, palm down. Move your hand up and down, trying to move your wrist through the greatest possible range of motion.

WRIST FLEXION Turn your palm up and repeat the above movements. Do fifty repetitions of this exercise, three times a day for three days. After three days, do the exercise with a three-pound dumbbell. As you get stronger, progress to a five- to six-pound weight; and if you really become powerful, use an eight-pound weight. To get the greatest benefit from these exercises, you must do them regularly and often.

Various companies make exercise devices that strengthen forearm muscles. Nautilus makes a small portable unit that is inexpensive and lets you select the resistance because one arm is working against the other.

Injuries to the Shoulders, Arms, and Hands   **149**

•After the early stages of the problem, which usually persist for one to two weeks, you can use heat in combination with ice. Anti-inflammation medication prescribed by your physician may be effective. Aspirin may also help. Chronic problems may be helped by a physical therapist who could use such therapy as ultrasound and electrical stimulation.

•Work to increase the strength of your arms and shoulders (see shoulder exercises, page 134, and arm exercises, pages 148, 149, and 151).

•Change your playing habits. This may include changing your techniques. Consult a good tennis pro who can teach you techniques that will place less strain on your elbow. Learn good mechanics and a smooth, relaxed stroke. During the early stages of recovery, try to cut down on your amount of play. Quit when you get tired. Fatigue can foster sloppy body mechanics that will only make your injury worse. Decrease the number of hours per session and the number of days you're playing. Rather than play every day, play every other day. Use the extra time to develop your strength, flexibility, and endurance.

•Examine your equipment. If you're playing with a heavy wooden racquet, change to something lighter and more flexible. Try to increase your grip size. A good tennis shop can help you choose appropriate equipment.

•Wear a tennis elbow brace. The brace fits around the thickest part of your forearm. Apply the brace firmly, but not so tight that it interferes with circulation. Adhesive tape will work just as well as a brace. Wrap the tape around the thickest part of your forearm. Remember, firm, but not tight.

•Severe tennis elbow may require medical help and in some cases surgery. However, in most cases, you can deal with this problem with the

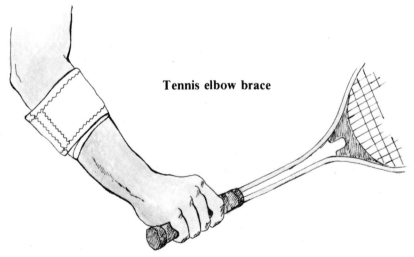

Tennis elbow brace

proper combination of rest, ice, strength and flexibility exercises, development of good technique, and selection of correct equipment.

Arm Exercises

The best exercises for tennis elbow are wrist extension and flexion and forearm supination and pronation (see page 148). General strengthening of arm and shoulder muscles may also be beneficial.

Biceps curls

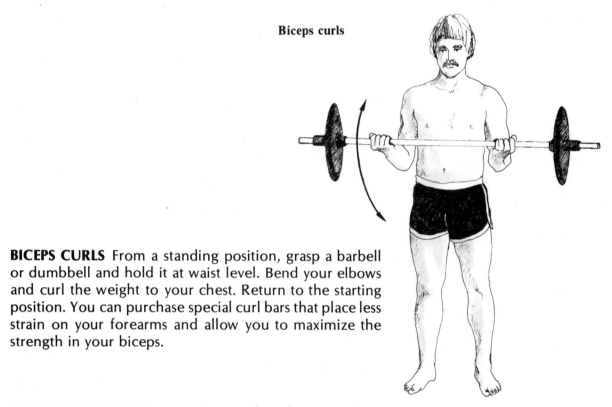

BICEPS CURLS From a standing position, grasp a barbell or dumbbell and hold it at waist level. Bend your elbows and curl the weight to your chest. Return to the starting position. You can purchase special curl bars that place less strain on your forearms and allow you to maximize the strength in your biceps.

ELBOW EXTENSIONS Lay supine on a bench, supporting a weight above your chest with elbows locked. Without moving your upper arms, bend your elbows and lower the weight behind your head. Press the weight to the starting position.

TENNIS BALL SQUEEZE Grasp a tennis ball or sponge rubber ball and squeeze. Carry the ball around with you and squeeze it periodically during the day.

Little League Elbow and Shoulder

These conditions are characterized by separations of the bone growth centers in the elbow or shoulder. The symptom is pain. They are caused by throwing a baseball too much. Little League elbow and shoulder have generated a great deal of misunderstanding and in some circles have resulted in creating a bad reputation for Little League baseball. The Little League has set up rules to limit the amount of pitching a player can do. These limits are well within the bounds of safety. Unfortunately, many children often do a considerable amount of pitching on their own, outside official practice. It's the extra strain of the outside practice that seems to cause the problems.

The curve ball had been considered the leading culprit in these injuries, but present scientific evidence indicates that this isn't the case. It's the amount of pitching, not the type of pitch that causes the problems. The curve ball takes more practice to learn than a fast ball, so in that respect, it's involved in the injury. If young players limit their amount of throwing, the chances of their getting these injuries are minimal. When the injury occurs, rest is essential. A player's prolonged participation when he or she has this condition could lead to problems later in life and perhaps hamper further athletic development.

Injuries to the Wrist

Injuries to the wrist in recreational sports occur most frequently in falls during activities such as basketball, skiing, and volleyball, and from exceeding the wrist's normal range of motion in sports such as weight lifting. Any wrist injury from a fall that causes pain that doesn't disappear after ten minutes should be evaluated by x-ray. There are numerous incidents in which people who had broken wrists delayed treatment for weeks because they thought the injury was a sprain. Treat all injuries of this nature as a break—seek medical attention.

In weight lifting, holding heavy weights in your hands with your wrists bent back in a hyperextended position can also result in wrist pain. This injury can be prevented by wearing leather wrist braces. This is an overuse injury and requires rest. Try to perform lifts that place less strain on your wrist. In general, the treatment for weight lifter's wrists is the same as for other sprains.

Treat a sprained wrist as follows:

• As with other soft tissue injuries, sprained wrists should be initially treated with ice, compression with an elastic bandage, and elevation.

• Any but the mildest wrist injuries should be evaluated by an x-ray examination.

• In the absence of fracture, you should attempt to maintain the range of motion. First, move your wrist forward and backward (flexion and extension). Next, move your wrist from side to side (abduction and adduction). Then circle your wrist clockwise and counterclockwise (circumduction). Icing your wrist before your exercises will help.

• As the pain begins to dissipate, begin wrist strengthening exercises. Perform wrist extension and flexion exercises (page 149) and the exercises below.

WRIST ROLLERS Find a cylindrical piece of wood and drill a hole through the middle of it. Tie one end of a length of rope through the hole in the wood and tie a weight on the other end. Turn the wood and roll up the rope.

DUMBBELL WRIST CIRCLES These also help strengthen wrist motions. Get an adjustable dumbbell and remove the center sleeve. Attach all of the weight at one end of the bar and grasp the other end. Make wrist circles—first clockwise, then counterclockwise. Gradually increase the amount of weight you're using.

Wrist rollers

●You can support your wrist with a simple taping application (overlap three lengths of tape around your wrist) or a leather brace. Elastic bandages available at sports stores provide little or no support. Other than for weight lifting, braces are no substitute for strong, flexible muscles.

Injuries to the Hands

Hand injuries are common in many sports. They range in severity from cuts and scrapes to loss of fingers. Any hand injury should be handled with great care because of the importance of your hands in your daily life. A loss of function can be devastating on many levels, so conservative treatment is essential. Injuries to this area can be extremely complex. A severed tendon in a finger for example, if treated early, can be easily repaired, but if left for only a week can curl up in the palm and be extremely difficult to deal with. Any injury to the hands, other than relatively minor ones, should be evaluated by a physician.

Scrapes, Cuts, Punctures, and Bites

The hands are susceptible to a variety of sudden traumatic injuries because of their importance in sports. Puncture wounds should be cleaned thoroughly and looked at by a physician to avoid the possibility of infection. Human bites to the hand can occur rather innocently, such as by striking someone's tooth in a basketball game, and can be potentially dangerous. Approximately 10 percent of human bites on the finger have resulted in amputations. Great care should be taken to clean the area and a physician should be consulted to administer antibiotics. Scrapes and cuts should be well cleaned and bandaged. Blisters on the hands should be treated like those on the feet. If the blister is broken, clean and protect the area. If the blister isn't broken, insert a sterile needle at it's base, drain it, then clean and dress the area.

Strains and Sprains of the Hands

These injuries are common in many sports. They can occur if you fall on an outstretched hand or if your fingers are bent back when you're trying to catch a ball; or they can occur as a result of overuse in such sports as golf or gymnastics.

The majority of sudden traumatic injuries of this nature should be evaluated by x-ray examination. Wrist and hand sprains range in severity from mild—involving pain but little tissue damage, to serious—involving partial or complete tearing of ligaments and tendons.

The initial treatment for strains and sprains involves ice, compression, and elevation. Apply an ice pack to the area and wrap it with an ace bandage. Try to maintain range of motion in the area. You can do this by simply opening and closing your hand. For strength development and continued rehabilitation, the best exercise is to squeeze a rubber ball.

Fingernail Injuries

Blood can collect under the fingernail if your fingernails are banged forcefully on a hard object such as a water ski. This injury can be extremely painful. Icing your fingers immediately for fifteen to thirty minutes and for several days after the injury will do much to relieve pain.

Injuries Caused by Wearing Rings

Ring injuries in sports are senseless and easily avoided. You should never wear rings or other jewelry when you're involved in physical activity. It's easy to catch a ring on a fence, net, or basket hoop. When a ring gets caught on something, your finger is asked to support a lot of weight all at once. The result can be massive damage to tissue, nerves, and blood vessels that may not be reparable. These injuries are often extremely serious and can result in amputation of a finger.

Instant Replay

●Prevention of shoulder and arm pain requires muscular strength, flexibility, and endurance.

●Good techniques are essential. Learn to use your whole body and not just your arms in upper body sports.

●Purchase the appropriate equipment. For tennis, buy a racquet with the correct weight, flexibility, string tension, and grip size.

●Generally, the initial treatment for soft tissue injuries of the shoulder and arms is ice, compression, and elevation. Although you should cut down on vigorous play after these injuries, you should begin almost immediately to maintain normal range of motion.

●Treat all traumatic wrist injuries as bone breaks and seek medical attention. Likewise, hand injuries can be devastating if not treated early and properly.

7.

GENERAL ACHES AND PAINS

In spite of our technologically advanced society that provides us with the finest medical care, instant communications, lifetime educational opportunities, and synthetic football fields, man is still a fragile animal in a hostile environment. We are subject to the heat and cold of the elements, animals that bite and sting us, and microscopic organisms that make us sick. Our bodies can fail us. If we try to avoid interacting with our environment by remaining inactive, we get fat and out of shape and subject ourselves to deterioration. If we gallantly sally forth to challenge the world, we get tennis elbow. There is no way that we are going to experience a pain-free existence—all we can do is watch out for the obvious and postpone the inevitable. With a little savvy and preparation, we can keep those aches and pains to a minimum.

Injuries to the Skin

Because of its extremely large surface area, your skin is easily injured in sports and physical activity. Usually the injuries are relatively benign. However, because of the danger of infection, always make sure that they are cared for properly.

Cuts, Scrapes, and Punctures

Breaks in the skin fall into four categories:

- Cuts
- Abrasions
- Punctures
- Lacerations

A cut is a penetration of the skin by a sharp edge. In recreational sports you can accidently get cut rather easily by doing such things as stepping on broken glass with bare feet. An abrasion occurs when the outer layer of skin is rubbed off—the resulting injury is called a strawberry. I got a beauty of an abrasion when I was skiing in California in June several years ago. In the warm weather I wasn't wearing a shirt, and when I fell at the top of a particularly steep pitch, I slid down the hill on my belly. The icy, granular spring snow felt like sandpaper. Needless to say, I deposited much of my outer shell on the slope—now I know how snakes feel when they shed their skin. A puncture occurs when your skin is penetrated by a sharp, pointed object such as a knife or nail. This injury occurs in a variety of circumstances, some typical—like stepping on a nail—some odd. I once saw a young teenaged boy who got a puncture wound playing baseball. He was striding into third base when his switchblade knife opened in his back pocket, creating a nasty puncture wound. A laceration is a tearing of the skin that can occur by catching your hand on a fence or someone's tooth.

In general, treatment is similar for all of these skin injuries. You can stop any bleeding by applying pressure directly over the wound with a clean bandage or cloth. If you have difficulty arresting the bleeding, call a doctor. Clean the area thoroughly with soap and water. Apply a clean bandage over the wound, change it regularly, and look for signs of infection. Abrasions should be kept moist with petroleum jelly applied to the wound. Consult a physician if the wound is a puncture or is a cut over one inch long which has penetrated several layers of skin. In any of these situations, look for signs of infection: the wound will typically become painful to touch and will turn red; the injured area may become swollen as may your lymph glands which are located in your neck, groin, and armpits; you may get a fever and feel generally awful. These signs may manifest themselves anywhere from one to seven days after the injury.

Contamination of a skin wound can result in tetanus, also called lockjaw, a disease resulting in convulsions and fever. You can get a tetanus shot that will provide protection against this disease. It's a good idea to get this shot before you need it. If you sustain an injury in the mountains or on the desert, you may not have ready access to medical assistance.

Cosmetics should be considered when you sustain an injury to the skin. An improperly treated cut on your face can leave a permanent scar. That might not be so bad if you're a German duke showing off your last sword fight, but it may prevent you from winning any more beauty contests. If you get a facial cut, see a physician unless you know all about butterfly bandages.

Sunburn

The sun is your enemy. Prolonged exposure to its rays over a period of many years can lead to permanent damage to your skin—your skin can become irreversibly dry, wrinkled, and leatherlike. In some instances you can get skin cancer.

Lying out in the sun trying to change your skin color is a lot like

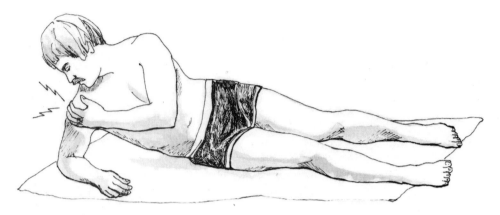

Sunburn can be a serious injury.

beating on your leg with a stick—both cause tissue damage. Now don't get me wrong, I love playing out in the sun, but if you are going to be exposed to sunlight for a prolonged period of time, protect yourself. Acquire your tan gradually and conservatively. Wear a good sunscreen and reapply it often when swimming or exercising.

Sunburn is caused by prolonged exposure to the ultraviolet rays of the sun. You start feeling it about two to eight hours after exposure. It actually kills skin cells and in some cases can damage skin blood vessels. Although dark skin color or a tan can help prevent sunburn, no one is immune to this problem. Some people burn more easily than others—if you are susceptible to sunburn, beware. Use a sunscreen and tan gradually and conservatively.

Different environments affect your chances of getting burned. At high altitudes the atmosphere is thinner, so more ultraviolet rays get through. If you couple high altitude with snow, you have to be extra careful. Snow reflects most light so you get the sun's rays directly from the sun and from the reflection off the snow. Spring is the time of greatest danger to the skier. The sun is out longer than in winter, so there is longer exposure. Mirror sunglasses, so stylish these days, can cause severe facial sunburn—the rays are reflected to the nose. Water can make for other problems. It can be deceiving—when you're in the water you feel cool, but the sun keeps cooking you. Eighty-five percent of the ultraviolet rays penetrate water three feet below the surface. In additon, beads of water on the skin act to focus the sunlight on your skin. The journal *The Physician and Sports Medicine* and the American Cancer Society have published some suggestions for safe sunning.

•Sun yourself before 10 a.m. and after 3 p.m. when ultraviolet rays are weakest. Limit your exposure at other times to short periods (ten to twenty minutes). Fair-skinned persons must be particularly careful about this.

•It is possible to get burned through light, casual clothes, especially during lengthy exposure to the sun. A beach umbrella does not offer full protection because ultraviolet rays are only partially deflected by it, and the rays bounce toward you from all directions—off sand, water, or other surfaces.

•A cloudy or foggy day can deceive the sunseeker, who might feel it would be safe to stay out longer. At least 70 percent of the burning power of the sun's rays penetrates the clouds, and persons who stay out for long periods can get severe burns.

•Water droplets or greasy preparations (such as baby oil) on the skin can cause a "lens effect," funneling the sun's rays onto the skin.

•Very effective screening lotions are those that contain PABA (para-aminobenzoic acid), which absorbs much of the ultraviolet rays but allows gradual tanning. Ask your physician or pharmacist about preparations that contain PABA. However, no lotion or cream will speed up tanning.

•Certain medications taken consistently can make you very sensitive to sunlight. These drugs include some diuretics (water pills), sulfonamides (combat infections), antibiotics, and tranquilizers. If you are taking medicine on a long-term basis, check with your physician before starting out to get a tan.

•Finally, remember that the sun is the leading cause of skin cancer. Anyone can develop skin cancer (there are 300,000 cases in the United States each year), but those who have fair or ruddy complexions and who are exposed to a great amount of sun, get it most often. Fortunately, 95 percent of skin cancer can be cured. Early warning signs for skin cancer include: a sore that does not heal, a change in the size or color of a wart or mole, or the development of any unusual pigmented (darkened) areas. As a rule of thumb, any skin change that persists should be brought to the attention of your physician.

Once you get a sunburn, try to avoid further exposure. Although this may ruin a vacation, it may also prevent skin problems that can last a long time. Start your treatment of your sunburn early. Taking aspirin every four hours is recommended by some dermatologists as a way of minimizing the inflammation. Anything you can do to lubricate your skin will help. An oil and ice compress is effective. Combine bath oil with four parts water; saturate a towel with this solution. Put the oily towel in crushed ice, then apply it to your sunburn.

Another remedy that's popular in tropical climates is to rub the juice from the leaves of an aloe plant on your sunburn. I first learned of this treatment from a ninety-year-old Hawaiian fisherman. At first I thought his advice was merely a folk remedy that wouldn't work. However, at the time my sunburn hurt so much, I was game for anything. The remedy worked wonders for me and now has gained acceptance among some physicians.

Cold Sores

Another skin problem that might be associated with exposure to the sun is cold sores caused by the herpes simplex virus. Cold sores, also called fever blisters, are small, painful open sores that form on the lips, nose, face, and genitalia. They can erupt due to a number of factors such as fatigue, cold, allergies, and emotional distress. They are common among skiers.

If you are prone to cold sores, try to protect the commonly affected areas. If you get them on your face, apply some protective cream before exposing yourself to the elements. A commonly used protective cream for skiers and lifeguards is zinc oxide. The only problem is that the protective cream can look worse than the problem you're trying to prevent. You'll look like you're auditioning for the Ringling Brothers Circus. There are other preparations available such as Glacier cream that look better yet still protect.

There are many commercially available medicines to combat cold sores. Researchers at Stanford Medical School have found a preparation of ether and chloroform to be effective in combating cold sores and preventing their further occurrence. Your doctor may be able to provide you with information about this remedy.

Mosquito Bites

The saying "don't bug me" has its origins dating from early campers and backpackers who ventured into mosquito-infested areas. Mosquito bites cause skin irritation and can make an otherwise enjoyable trip into the wild miserable. You can prevent the problem to a certain extent by applying insect repellent to your skin and clothing. When you're exercising, apply the repellent often because your sweating will cause much of it to disappear.

Ice helps to relieve some of the minor inflammation of mosquito bites as does calamine lotion. Another remedy is to apply meat tenderizer mixed in water directly over the bite.

Stings

Stings by bees, wasps, hornets, and yellow jackets are common whenever you exercise outdoors. The sting is accompanied by venom from the insect and can be pretty painful. Some people are allergic to stings—the results can be serious illness or death. If you are allergic to bee stings, you should have ready access to antibee venom that's available from your doctor.

If you get a bee sting, remove the stinger with tweezers and clean the area thoroughly with soap and water. If a severe reaction develops, seek medical attention immediately. Avoid bee stings by wearing shoes when you play on grass fields.

Frostbite

When you get frostbite, your tissue actually freezes. The condition is serious; you should try your best to prevent it. It's somewhat common among skiers who go out on very cold, windy days without adequate protection for the face or hands. To treat frostbite experts recommend placing the frostbitten body part in water heated to 100–108°F until the tissue is thawed. Use a thermometer to keep the water within this temperature range—if the water temperature rises above 109°F, tissue damage may occur. After it is thawed the body part should be kept cool to lessen metabolism and assist in convalescence. Try to keep the frostbitten part covered. It's important to maintain circulation by keeping the body warm with blankets. See a physician as soon as possible.

Muscle Soreness

Muscle soreness is an overuse condition that may last for several days after exercise. It usually appears after exercise when you're out of shape or when you markedly increase the amount or intensity of your exercise program. Any time you stress a muscle in a new way, you risk muscle soreness. You could, for example, develop sore muscles hiking in the hills even though you run several miles every day. Walking up hills may place stress on your legs that isn't present during your daily jog.

A recent series of studies by Dr. William Abraham of the University of Rochester School of Medicine has shown that delayed muscle soreness is probably due to overstretching your muscle's elastic components. The elastic component is the connective tissue that holds the muscles together and gives them flexibility. When you exercise, you stress not only your muscles, but also the connective tissue that holds them together.

The causes of muscle soreness have been studied for almost eighty years—the topic remains extremely controversial. Other hypothesized causes of muscle soreness have included structural damage to muscle, muscle spasms, and lactic acid accumulation in muscles.

The best way to avoid muscle soreness is to avoid sudden and dramatic increases in your exercise. Increase the severity of your program gradually. Remember, injuries are almost always caused by exceeding the capacity of some part of your body. If your capacity is low, it doesn't take much of an overload to cause injury. Build up slowly.

Soreness can range in severity from very mild to extremely severe. You can become so sore that you can barely move. The treatment for soreness depends upon the severity. If you are extremely sore, you should treat the problem like a pulled muscle. Use ice massage and rest. Heat may make severe muscle soreness worse. If your whole body is sore, pick the parts of your body that are causing you the most misery. You can use heat for mild soreness. This shouldn't create any complications and will make you feel better. Static stretching of your sore muscle and range of motion exercises, particularly in a swimming pool or whirlpool bath, may also help you get rid of some of the pain. (Range of motion exercises for most areas of the body are described in Chapters 4 through 6.)

For reasons presently unknown, certain types of strenuous exercise do not cause muscle soreness. It is very rare that you would get sore after using some of the new isokinetic exercise machines such as the Cybex. These machines exercise your muscles at relatively fast speeds. It may be that with these machines forces sufficient to cause damage are never created within your muscles. Working a muscle through a full range of motion rather than a restricted range also seems to produce less soreness. So when you're weight training, for example, don't cheat and do only part of the exercise—you will be less likely to develop muscle soreness if you go through the whole procedure.

Environmental Distress

Your body has the ability to maintain a biological balance at a variety of extreme temperatures and environmental conditions. If it gets too hot, your body cools itself. If it gets too cold, your body gives you signals that it's time to seek shelter or put some more clothes on. If you're at high altitude, you automatically breathe harder to provide yourself with the necessary oxygen. These protective devices have their limits, however. You should be aware of these limitations so that you can enjoy sports safely in your present environment.

Altitude Sickness

Altitude sickness can occur in anyone who goes up high enough. Most people begin to experience the symptoms at about 11,000 feet, but the onset may occur anywhere from 6,000 to 15,000 feet.

Mary, a medical student visiting the Aspen State Teacher's College for a medical seminar, experienced a classic case of altitude sickness. I met her in the Paragon, one of Aspen's favorite watering holes. She looked ill—her head was bowed down, and she was staring into a glass of Perrier water.

"Hey baby, what's happening?" (My subtle approach.)

"Please leave me alone," she pleaded, "I'm not feeling very well."

"Listen, maybe I can help; what's the matter?"

In the typical condescending tone of a future physician, she exclaimed, "I've been experiencing headache, insomnia, irritability, vomiting, tachycardia, dyspnea, and general malaise. In addition, at night I've developed Cheyne–Stokes breathing patterns." (Translated, she said that she was feeling lousy, her heart was beating rapidly, her breathing was sometimes difficult and irregular, and she had no desire to be picked up in a bar. Little did she know, however, that I was writing a book on athletic injuries and could possibly help.)

"I have some suggestions—you are obviously suffering from altitude sickness. You should get some rest and try to breathe more slowly. The symptoms should disappear as you acclimatize to this altitude." (Aspen is at 9,200 feet.)

She followed my advice—when I saw her the next evening, she was much better and very grateful.

Usually altitude sickness disappears as you adjust to your new environment. When you first go to a high altitude, your breathing rate increases because the air is thinner. However, by breathing harder you lower the carbon dioxide level in your blood. This causes the blood vessels in your brain to constrict slightly, which causes some people to get sick. As you remain at high altitude, your body experiences several chemical adaptations that restore balance and your feeling of well-being. Sometimes, altitude sickness is accompanied by serious conditions: pulmonary and cerebral edema (fluid accumulation in your lungs and brain). When either of these conditions occur, you should seek medical attention or go to a lower altitude. These conditions usually occur only at extremely high altitudes.

If you are hiking and camping at altitude, there are several things you can do to minimize discomfort.

•Get in good physical condition before you venture to high altitude for hiking or skiing. Remember, above 6,000 feet your endurance capacity decreases about 3 percent for every one thousand feet you

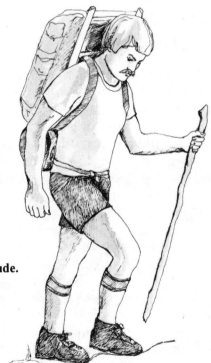

Being in good physical condition is the best preparation for a trip to high altitude.

go up. If you have a low exercise capacity, you will easily fatigue at high altitude.

•Avoid heavy exercise until you've had a chance to adjust to your new environment.

•If you're experiencing altitude sickness and irregular breathing at night while camping at high altitude, try sleeping with your head facing into your sleeping bag. This will cause you to rebreathe your own carbon dioxide and will greatly reduce your symptoms.

•Make sure you drink enough water. Exercising at high altitude can dehydrate you very easily—your sweat evaporates much faster because of the dry air and you lose a lot more body water through breathing.

•Protect yourself from the effects of the sun. You are much more susceptible to sunburn at high altitude because the air is thinner—more ultraviolet rays get through.

Dehydration and Heat-Related Problems

Your body can be described as a large column of fluid. It depends upon water to maintain an optimal internal environment. Not only is water necessary to facilitate the various chemical reactions that occur in your body, but it's vital for maintaining a constant body temperature when you exercise or are exposed to heat. Water loss of only 10 percent of body weight has caused death in some individuals. Adequate water intake is essential for good health and optimal exercise performance.

Most people don't drink enough water when they're exercising or are exposed to heat. You should get in the habit of taking water breaks. I've seen people lose five pounds during a jogging session or a heavy game of tennis. Ideally, you should replace lost water at regular intervals. This will have a significant effect on your exercise capacity and on the way you feel. Force yourself to drink a little more water than you want. A good rule of thumb for runners and those involved in heavy work is to attempt to drink about a half pint of water for every fifteen minutes of exercise. Increase this amount if it's hot outside.

Water is the best fluid replacement. Many of the commercially available fluid replacements are too high in sugar and electrolyte (sodium, potassium, magnesium, etc.). The high sugar content in some of these products slows down the time it takes for water to get into your system. The high electrolyte concentration can actually lead to a type of dehydration. To replace fluids, drink water—preferably cold water. It's cheap and it's the most effective.

Muscle cramps have been associated with insufficient amounts of electrolytes in the muscles. The classic treatment for cramps has been salt pills. Recent research, however, has shown salt pills to be ineffective. X-rays have shown that salt pills remain in the stomach practically intact for several hours after being consumed. Studies by Dr. David Costill, former president of the American College of Sports Medicine, have shown that your body has a remarkable ability to maintain electrolyte balance, and that it is the lack of fluid that you should be most concerned with. As long as the electrolyte content in your diet is adequate, you need no additional supplements like salt pills. If you feel you must consume commercial fluid replacements, drink them after exercise—drink water during exercise.

Many people try to cool themselves during exercise by toweling themselves with a wet cloth. This procedure is of only limited benefit. What will do you the most good when you exercise in the heat is drinking a lot of water. With a little practice, you will be able to tolerate this easily.

You should learn to recognize the symptoms of dehydration and thermal distress. If you begin to feel a throbbing pressure in your temples and a cold sensation over your upper body, your body temperature may be getting too high. The best thing to do is to stop exercising and cool your body down gradually—drink a lot of water and rest in a cool place. If your symptoms are severe, see a physician immediately.

Thermal distress can manifest itself in a number of ways. Heat stroke is the most serious type of heat-related injury. In this condition, your biological thermostat, the hypothalamus, loses its ability to regulate your body temperature. Rapid cooling is essential or you may die from heat stroke. Heat exhaustion is another problem encountered. Heat exhaustion is a condition in which you don't have enough blood to meet your body's demands. During exercise in the heat, blood is needed by your working muscles and by your skin. Your total blood volume may be inadequate to meet the needs of all of these tissues. Your blood pressure may fall and your system may not be pumping enough blood and oxygen to your brain—you may faint. The best treatment is to lie down in a cool place with your feet elevated.

It takes time to acclimatize to the heat. As with exposure to altitude, body adaptation to hot environments occurs, but it occurs gradually. You can facilitate the process by becoming physically fit; fitness speeds up heat acclimatization. You can help yourself adapt by progressively increasing the amount of exercise you perform in the heat. Exercise seems to be required to maximally acclimatize to heat.

The clothing you wear during exercise is important in preventing thermal distress. You should avoid wearing heavy sweat shirts if there is any danger of overheating yourself. On hot days, wear light clothing that allows for heat dissipation. Many running shirts produced today are vented to allow for the evaporation of sweat.

Avoid rubber exercise suits like the plague. These garments make you lose a lot of weight—water weight. Remember that dehydration and thermal distress are highly correlated. When you want to lose weight, lose fat not water. Your body's water balance is delicate. Water losses are quickly compensated for after you consume fluids. Weight loss in the form of dehydration is an exercise in futility and is potentially dangerous.

Smog

Exercising on a smoggy day may cause respiratory distress. When you exercise you naturally breathe harder, and thus you tend to take in more smog into your lungs. Smog, unfortunately, is part of urban life. It is undoubtedly a contributor to various types of cancer and lung disease. Unless you plan to move to a smogless environment, you've got to learn to live with it. A healthy respiratory system that's capable of a high level of function can adequately clear pollution products from your system. Regular endurance exercise, such as running, swimming, or cycling, done on a regular basis, is necessary for a healthy cardio-respiratory system. It's better to be fit than unfit—whether there is smog or not.

It's probably better not to exercise during a heavy smog alert. High levels of the primary pollutants—carbon monoxide, sulfur dioxide, ozone, and nitrogen dioxide—will decrease your performance and make breathing difficult. If you're a smoker, the problem is compounded. Smog levels are usually lower early in the morning and late at night. If it's smoggy, try to avoid training during commuter hours.

If you've exercised too heavily on a smoggy day and have a tight feeling in your lungs, try to lie down in a cool place and relax. Rest will help you to slow down your breathing. If your breathing problems are serious, see your doctor.

Motion Sickness

Motion sickness can occur in sports such as sailing, fishing, and river rafting. The cause of this problem is excessive stimulation of the balance center in your inner ear (vestibular apparatus). The primary symptoms are nausea and vomiting. Although motion sickness is known by many names—air sickness, car sickness, river-raft sickness—the cause for each is exactly the same. You may be more susceptible to the problem at certain times than at others. If you tend to get one type of motion sickness, you are just as prone to other types as well.

Emotional factors can play a part. I was Marlin fishing in Hawaii on a day when the ocean was particularly rough. For six hours we bobbed about in waves that seemed to toss the boat around in several directions at once. Everyone on board was feeling a little queasy. All of a sudden we hit a giant fish—excitement radiated through the boat. I immediately snapped out of my motion sickness, even though the water wasn't any calmer.

If you are susceptible to motion sickness, you should take steps to minimize discomfort before the problem arises. Over-the-counter medications, such as Bonine, can be effective if taken before the boat ride or plane trip. Try to minimize ascending motion as much as possible. Sit in the middle of the boat or over the wings in a plane. Try to avoid reading or watching the rolling horizon. Avoid alcohol or big meals before exposure to motion. You are better off, however, if you have a light meal several hours before exposure.

Sickness and Exercise

Today's casual athlete is extremely serious—sometimes too serious. You shouldn't feel guilty if you miss some training time because of illness. Examine the reason you've been training in the first place: exercise makes you healthier, makes you look better, and makes you feel better; and, exercise is fun. If you try to train when you're sick, you are violating all of the basic assumptions of your exercise program—you'll run the risk of getting sicker, you'll look like hell, and you won't have fun.

Exercising when you're sick isn't very smart. Viral infections are sometimes associated with myocarditis, an inflammation of the heart. Doctors agree that exercise is bad for you when you have myocarditis. This condition can lead to heart damage and, in some cases, death. If you have the flu or an illness with a fever, don't exercise until at least several days after the symptoms are gone. As a rule of thumb, rest one day for every day you were sick before resuming your program. When you start again, exercise at a lower intensity. Let exercise improve your health—

not make it worse. Don't let your exercise program cause you to *get* sick either. Take some simple precautions. Don't overtrain; condition yourself gradually and avoid extreme fatigue. Eat a sensible diet that contains an adequate amount of carbohydrates. Don't let your muscles get chilled after exercise—put on a sweat shirt and stay warm. Avoid too much emotional stress—relax and enjoy sports.

Gastrointestinal Distress

Indigestion and gas pains can disturb your exercise performance and feeling of well-being during sports. The two main causes of these problems are the food you eat and, to a certain extent, emotional distress. Eat slowly, try to avoid irritating foods, and try to eat smaller portions at your meals. You can avoid stomach problems by restricting your pre-exercise meals to foods that are easy to digest. These meals should be light and low in fats and protein. Avoid the classic pregame steak dinner. This meal takes a long time to digest and tends to sit in your stomach for a long time.

Irregular Menstruation

Irregular menstruation has become a rather common phenomenon among women involved in endurance exercise, such as distance running and swimming. A survey conducted by Dr. Ken Foreman of Seattle Pacific University indicates that this condition is common among women involved in particularly vigorous training programs. This phenomenon seems to be related to a critical level of body fat. Women who drop below 16 percent fat seem to experience irregular menstrual periods. (The average percentage of body fat for women is between 20 and 25 percent.) The body may interpret the abnormally low fat levels as a type of starvation—a period not very conducive to a healthy pregnancy. Young female endurance athletes typically experience late menarche (first menstruation). When they cease competing, menarche occurs. This delay in menarche is certainly consistent with the critical fat percentage hypothesis. Dr. Harmon Brown, U.S. women's track and field team physician, has stated that the effects of exercise-related menstrual irregularity on health are not known. At this time, I wouldn't recommend distance running as a viable form of birth control.

Pregnancy, Exercise, and Athletic Injuries

Athletic injuries, and for that matter, exercise in general, have not been studied very much in pregnant women. However, there are several factors that should be considered. Pregnancy greatly affects your center of gravity—the pelvic tilt changes and the curve of the lower back becomes greater. These changes in themselves make you more prone to injuries and various aches and pains—particularly back trouble. Another pregnancy-related change is that the joints seem to lose some of their stability possibly due to an increase in the secretion of the hormone relaxin which has a direct effect upon connective tissue. It is not known whether there is any relationship between an increased joint laxity and injury during pregnancy. You should seek specific advice from your obstetrician before beginning an exercise program.

Current research indicates that exercise and fitness are beneficial for both the mother and the baby. But because of center of gravity changes and possible increased susceptibility to joint injury, it's a good idea to choose sports and exercises carefully. It's probably best to restrict your training to exercises that don't require rapid changes of direction. An excellent exercise during pregnancy is swimming. Swimming offers the beneficial effects of training on your cardiovascular system and muscles, but doesn't subject you too much to the effects of gravity. Walking also provides an excellent form of exercise during pregnancy. Jogging is practiced by many pregnant women. This form of exercise may possibly affect implantation during the first few months of pregnancy. However, if you are used to running, in most cases, you should be able to continue this activity with little difficulty.

Dr. Hugh Bonner, an exercise physiologist from the University of Texas, has found that exercise by the mother during pregnancy will increase the strength of the heart of the newborn. This could possibly result in a heart that has a higher pumping capacity. Studies have shown that exercise by the mother should not be exhaustive but around 60–80 percent of maximal capacity.

Obesity and Injuries

In addition to its role as a risk factor of coronary heart disease, obesity can increase your chances of receiving an athletic injury. Excess weight compounds the forces acting on vulnerable joints. In addition, your excess weight will accentuate the effects of an existing injury by exerting a lot more pressure on an injured part. Fortunately, exercise exerts a positive force on a weight control program. With a consistent effort to reduce caloric intake and increase caloric expenditure, you may be able to reduce body fat and with it, the risk of injury. If you are overweight, you should begin your exercise program with activities such as walking, cycling, or swimming, rather than running. Running may place stresses on your joints that may easily result in an injury. You can consider making running your exercise as you become better conditioned.

Instant Replay

- When you get a skin wound, clean the area thoroughly and watch for infection.
- Protect your skin against the sun. Tan gradually and use sunscreens.
- Muscle soreness is an overuse condition that is caused by doing too much exercise too soon. The physiological causes are not completely understood.
- Adjust to higher altitudes gradually. Don't begin heavy exercise in the mountains until you have at least partially acclimatized.
- The best fluid replacement is water. Drink water regularly during exercise in the heat.
- If you live in a smoggy area, exercise in spite of the polluted environment. Avoid training during periods of the day when pollution is greatest (commuter hours).
- Prevent motion sickness before it occurs. Some over-the-counter medications such as Bonine are effective if taken before exposure to motion. Avoid alcohol and large meals before going on a boat, raft, etc.
- Menstrual irregularity has been reported by women involved in heavy endurance exercise. This may be related to reduced body fat. The relationship of this phenomenon to health is unknown at present.

INDEX